Growing Taller Secrets
Second Edition

*Journey Into The World
Of Human Growth And Development*

Robert Grand

Atlantic Business Communications - New York, NY
2010

Growing Taller Secrets: *Journey Into The World of Human Growth and Development* / Robert Grand - 2nd Edition

Published by:
Atlantic Business Communications Inc.
1375 Broadway New York, NY 10018

P. cm.

ISBN - 13: 978-0-9677655-2-5
ISBN - 10: 0-9677655-2-8

1. Human growth.   2. Physical and mental exercise.   3. Diet.   I. Title

DISCLAIMER:

Any person with a serious health problem should seek treatment from their health care professional.

This information is not intended to replace the advice of your physicians. Those already undergoing physician-prescribed therapy should neither stop taking, nor reduce the dosage of such treatment without their physician's directions.

These statements have not been evaluated by the U.S. Food & Drug Administration, and are not intended to diagnose, treat, cure or prevent any disease.

Always consult a nutritionist, dietitian, licensed medical practitioner and professionally certified personal trainer prior to taking any supplement, modifying your diet and/or beginning any exercise program.

This book is dedicated to my beautiful and smart children, my true soulmate wife, my genius sister, my mentors parents, my big family, and my great friends. Most of all, it is dedicated to you, my reader – the self-made superstar of tomorrow.

Contents

Can I Grow Taller?

Dear friend, if you are holding this book in your hands – there must be a good reason for it: most likely you or your loved one needs help. Let me say it straight from the start: the only person who can really help you in your need is yourself. Only you can accomplish what you have ever wanted! Only you can increase your height to the limit of your potential. All you need is willingness, persistence, knowledge and belief in your success. Willingness and persistence I cannot provide to you, while the knowledge and belief in your success – I can. In this book, I will give you all the knowledge you will ever need to gain you height. I will also give you some other extremely important clues and secrets following which will help you to succeed not only in your physical growth, but also in your personal growth (whatever you think it is), for the rest of your life!

Very important: don't start reading this book from the end or the middle. **Start from the beginning and do not skip anything** because all information I am giving you is important even if you may think it is not (well, you may probably skip the list of growth disorders in the next chapter).

There are probably lots of big questions in your mind: Is it actually possible to affect the growth of my body and grow taller? Will I ever be gaining at least a little to my current height? How tall will I be till next summer? How tall will I be when I stop growing? When will I stop growing? Will this book help me? Will it be hard to affect my growth? How soon will I see any results?

My goal, my dear friend, is not only to give you answers to all or most of your questions, but also to help you actually accomplish great deal in your goals whatever they might be, including growing taller.

I will not get into big discussion of why you or anyone else would want to be taller. It is just part of the human nature to be wanted, to be respected, and it is easier in most cases to gain respect of others in the beginning of any relationship if you are equally tall or taller. Why do you think in almost any TV program a host of the program sits higher than others? Because they hope to gain more respect from the audience or people they are interviewing by looking down at them. It is natural for a person to feel more important when he looks down at someone, and less important – when looks up.

> *Don't get me wrong; it is not that hard to get around this without even growing taller. All you have to do is think BIG, think that you only appear shorter but feel much taller than people surrounding you. Trust me, that thought alone may change your appearance in ways you could never imagine.*

Have you ever had the experience of meeting a person that is shorter than you are, and your first impression was – real respect? I bet you did. For some strange reason the person you have never met before caught your attention in a good way regardless of his height or weight, sometimes even without saying a word. There is a simple explanation to this: every one of us releases energy that is created by our thoughts. We cannot see this energy, but we can feel it. That is the energy that you felt when you met that person and unintentionally reacted with positive impression (it can often be negative too). How did that person do it? Most likely he does not know anything about this energy of thought, he just thinks BIG, he respects himself and others, he knows firmly that he can accomplish anything, and he expects people to respect him the way he is. Not only you, anyone who meets that person will feel respect towards him, not even noticing how tall or short he is.

Later on we will get into more details on energy of your thought – you will need it as a very important part of your quest to grow taller, but I will just say that the person that people feel good about and respect even at the first sight, regardless of his height, can easily be you. ***Just take what you just read seriously, and you will be surprised how well it works.***

As much as I believe that you can do just fine with the height you already have, whatever it is, I also believe that if you can increase your height – you should. Yes, you may make you life a little easier being taller. Yes, it feels better to look people straight or down into their eyes, not up. Moreover, if you will gain your height by following my program and my advices, you will not only be taller, but also much better-off with your health and personal growth for the rest of your life. I'm not exaggerating.

To answer you big question of how successful will you be in increasing your height, I will repeat myself by saying that it depends on your willingness and persistence. However, I will give you some general rules and statistics, which may not necessarily apply to you, but will give you some ideas of what your chances are and how much more you can grow.

The general pace of gaining height for most children between the ages of 3 and early adolescence is about 2 inches (5 cm) per year. It can definitely fluctuate. No one grows with the constant pace. In years of early adolescence, for example, sex hormones often contribute to a much faster growth rate. Different time of the year also shows different growth rates, such as late spring and summer is time when children are generally growing faster than in the fall and winter. By the way, why do you think late spring and summer are so height productive? Because during these periods we unintentionally do more right things for the body to grow faster. When you will finish reading this book, you will understand exactly what I mean.

Under normal circumstances, the age at which we stop growing fluctuate very substantially. Girls are almost always stop growing earlier than boys, on average 3 – 4 years earlier, which happens anywhere between ages of 14 and 21. Boys stop growing anywhere between ages of 17 and 25. Please also understand that ***these age limits can be increased by up to 3 to 5 more years of growth for boys and girls if they do something about this, which this book is all about.***

Those are statistics, but what about me – you would ask. It is impossible to tell when you will stop growing, however there are several factors you can use to give yourself a clue.

The **first factor** is **when your puberty begins,** which is usually between ages of 8 and 13 for girls, 10 and 15 for boys. The later your puberty begins – the later you stop growing. By the way, during first two years from when the puberty starts it is normal to expect a very active growth spurt for boys and girls. At this time they can gain as much as 3 to 5 inches (7 cm – 12 cm) per year.

The **second factor** is our **genetics**. Let me try to explain it as simply as I can. Our body is a combination of trillions of cells, each containing the same molecule that carries the complete set of instructions for making all the proteins a cell will ever need. This molecule is called DNA, which is a combination of different genes (microscopic particles each containing instructions for a particular protein). These genes were inherited to us from our past generations through our parents and will be inherited from us to our children and future generations. Genes are responsible for the likeliness we have to our parents and close relatives because we share great number of them. Genes give our body instructions on how it should be developed. At the same time, those instructions are more like directions or suggestions and are not "written in stone". It means that you are an architect of not only your destiny but also your body. As you can see, it is also impossible to predict your final height based on genetics, however looking at your parents and close relative's average heights will give you an idea how tall you may be, especially if your parents and relatives are of similar heights.

A simple way to calculate the average probable final height of a person is as follows:

$$((1.58 + 0.15) + 1.75)) / 2 = 1.74 \text{ cm}$$

For men – add 6 inches (15 cm) to their mother's height, then average it out with father's height: ((mother's height + 6″) + father's height) / 2.

For women – subtract 6 inches (15 cm) from their father's height, then average it out with mother's height ((father's height – 6″) + mother's height) / 2.

You should not be discouraged if everyone in your family is short. If you have enough time before you stop growing, use this book as a guide – and you will have much greater chance of growing taller than anyone in your family. On the average, people who follow my program add 2 to 5 inches (5 – 13 cm) to their final height, often even more, sometimes much more. **The earlier you start – the more you will gain.**

> *If you are trying to figure out your possible final height based on your parents' height, one important question you should not miss – did your parents do everything right to be as tall as they could be when they were younger and still growing? Most people, likely including your parents, did not grow as much as they could simply because they and their parents did not know how to affect the body's growth. That is why it is very possible that your parents could be much taller would they do everything their body needed to grow taller. It means that calculating your possible final height based on your parents' height may be much less accurate than you would hope so.*

I suggest you to study this book thoroughly, understand every aspect of what makes the body grow, and then find out from your parents what they did or did not do correctly in their childhood (if they will remember) in comparison to what you will learn in this book. If you've learned that they've got many things wrong, and you still have enough time to grow, simply dismiss the above-mentioned probable final height formula because it is quite possible for you to grow much taller than both of your parents.

The ***third factor*** is **age.** If a person's puberty began 4 – 5 years ago, the pace of body's growth decreases substantially. It does not mean that a person in his late teens or early-mid twenties who follow this program is unlikely to grow. It means the growth rate will likely be slower and end result may not be as significant compared to a person who started to follow my advices earlier. You can also ask your doctor to take X-rays of bones and compare them with bone X-rays of an average person in your age. If a doctor finds that your bones look younger than what could be expected in your age, you have a constitutional growth delay, which usually is the result of delayed puberty. It means your bones will likely continue to develop for longer than you could expect.

The ***fourth factor*** is **how you were raised** during first years of life. You should understand that there are number of factors that not you, but your parents had control over since the moment of your conception. We will discuss all of them in detail later in the book, but some of them are: if a mother was drinking, smoking, had a lot of stress, had poor nutrition or incorrect diet during pregnancy or while breastfeeding, if during first years of life a child receives not enough of necessary nutrition, but a lot of junk food, is not physically active, rarely allowed to be exposed to direct sunlight and fresh air, get sick a lot, the future final height of a child may be diminished by these factors. Another big factor is the weight of a baby at birth, as larger born babies tend to grow larger as adults.

The ***fifth factor*** is … well – **your knowledge, your belief and your actions**. Study this book and you will understand.

Growth Disorders

Most short children do not have serious growth problems. A child's rate of growth is an important clue to the presence or absence of a growth problem. If a child is growing at a much slower than normal rate, you should be aware that there are some diseases that can cause poor growth and the child should definitely be checked by a good doctor. Please understand, this book is not designed to help treat or prevent any diseases (even though all activities shown in this book may help to prevent many diseases), it designed to help healthy individuals to grow. That is why if you suspect or have any concern over your health, please discuss it with your doctor first.

There are several major disorders that affect body's growth such as disorders of endocrine system, growth hormone deficiency, turner syndrome, hypothyroidism and dwarfism.

Many **disorders of endocrine system**, which is made up of glands that produce hormones controlling the growth, are more common reasons for growth disorder.

Growth hormone deficiency is the condition when the pituitary gland (hypophysis), which is responsible for producing the growth hormone among others, does not produce enough hormones for the body to grow. It could happen for number of reasons, including tumors near pituitary gland, damaged hypothalamus or pituitary gland often at birth, by trauma or certain diseases.

Turner syndrome affects about 1 in every 2,500 girls due to a problem with their genes. Girls with Turner syndrome are born with only one X chromosome or they are missing part of one X chromosome, and often will never reach puberty and sexual maturity unless they get treatment for the condition such as growth hormone treatment or estrogen replacement. Girls with Turner syndrome are usually diagnosed either at birth or around the time they might be expected to go through puberty.

Hypothyroidism is a very common condition when the thyroid gland is not producing enough thyroid hormone, which runs the body's metabolism and also necessary to support normal growth.

Dwarfism is a medical condition characterized by extreme small size. Dwarfism can be caused by more than 200 different medical conditions; most are caused by a spontaneous genetic mutation in the egg or sperm cells prior to conception. Other conditions are caused by genes inherited from one or both parents. Some causes include metabolic or hormonal disorders in infancy or childhood.

There are other disorders that often affect human growth and need to be brought to the doctor's attention. Most of them are postural defects such as scoliosis, knee flexion, bowlegs and knock-knees. All of the activities described in this book should not worsen any of these conditions, and will possibly improve them. However you should consult a doctor on what physical activities you can do, what diet you can have and what is not recommended. Nevertheless, **before you go to the doctor, I strongly suggest finishing reading this book** because then you will know much more about what affects your body's growth, probably even more than your doctor, and will know what to ask and what to expect.

The program you are about to learn in this book includes physical activities that are not hard to follow, but if you are new to sports or exercise, or had an injury in the past that you think may have some impact on you, it will be a good idea to visit your physician before starting those physical activities. If you are physically active and have not had any prior injuries, you don't need a physical exam before you begin this program.

If your doctor is telling you that you are healthy, just destined to be short, and there is nothing to be done about it, don't believe him and read further.

Program basics
(and why you should believe in your success)

The program you will learn in this book consists of several main parts which are: **using power of thought to trigger growth**, **activities to increase growth hormone level**, **specially designed exercise program** that prepares muscles and stimulates joints for best results, **correct use of water, salt and sun** as very important components for your body's development, **correct breathing**, and **specially designed diet** to give your body everything it needs to grow taller.

Each part of the program by itself is powerful enough to give you some results, but the same part is much more powerful when used together with all other parts. We can compare this to a great tasting food recipe with lots of ingredients. If we don't include some of these ingredients, you may probably be able to eat that food, but it will not taste good. Another example – your body needs air, water and food to be able to live, and will not survive if one of these ingredients will not be supplied. Got the point?

Before you will learn what to do, **I want you to believe that height can be affected by many factors, not because I said so, but because there are many facts and studies that prove so.** Let me give you first of all some important excerpt from several different studies that will show you that *the height of a person can be controlled and depends on person's activities, the environment and the mindset*.

From the study "Determinants of variation in adult body height" by Karri Silventoinen, published in a Journal of Biosocial Science (2003), 35:2:263-285 Cambridge University Press: *"In modern Western societies, about 20% of variation in body height is due to environmental variation. In poorer environments, this proportion is probably larger, with lower heritability of body height as well as larger socioeconomic body height differences. The role of childhood environment is seen in the increase in body height during the 20th century simultaneously with the increase in the standard of living. The most important non-genetic factors affecting growth and adult body height are nutrition and diseases. Short stature is associated with poorer education and lower social position in adulthood. This is mainly due to family background, but other environmental factors in childhood also contribute to this association. Body height is a good indicator of childhood living conditions, not only in developing countries but also in modern Western societies."*

From the study "Early Life Factors Are Determinants of Female Height at Age 19 Years in a Population-Based Birth Cohort" (Pelotas, Brazil) by Denise P. Gigante, Bernardo L. Horta, Rosângela C. Lima, Fernando C. Barros, and Cesar G. Victora, published by American Society for Nutrition J. Nutr. (February 2006) 136:473-478, jn.nutrition.org: *"The most important nongenetic factors affecting growth and adult body height are nutrition and diseases". "Environmental factors, such as social class, parental education, maternal smoking during pregnancy, prenatal and postnatal growth have all been related to height". "Girls who belonged to poor families and whose mothers were in the lowest schooling category were 4 cm shorter than girls from rich families whose mothers had 9 y of schooling". "Girls whose mothers had smoked during pregnancy were 2 cm shorter than the others". "Adolescents who were stunted or underweight at age 2 or 4 y were 8 cm shorter at age 19 y". "Adolescents who were hospitalized during childhood were shorter than those who were not hospitalized".*

From the publication "Early environment and child-to-adult growth trajectories in the 1958 British birth cohort" by Leah Li, Orly Manor and Chris Power, published by American Journal of Clinical Nutrition (July 2004), 80:1:185-192, ajcn.org: *"Parental height, birth weight, maternal smoking during pregnancy, breastfeeding, parental divorce, and socioeconomic factors were all significantly associated with childhood height, but their effects differed thereafter. Parental height and birth weight were most strongly associated with offspring height, and their effects persisted". "Socioeconomic disadvantage (manual social class, large family size, and overcrowded households) was associated with substantial deficits of 2–3 cm (adjusted estimates) in height at 7 y. Catch-up growth was apparent but was insufficient to overcome the initial insult on growth". "Parental separation or divorce in the children's early life was significantly associated with height in childhood". "Boys whose parents divorced between ages 4 and 7 y were significantly shorter than their counterparts in childhood and in adulthood".*

As you can see, all these studies have much in common in their results. They all show that the environment plays a very important role in child's body growth, and the standard of living makes the biggest difference. Well, as we already discussed in the "forth factor" of human growth in the previous chapter, children who live in poverty usually get less nutrition then children from wealthy families, get sick more often and more serious, live with more problems and stress, all of which tremendously affect physical development and growth. It all means one thing – if you believe that some things do actually negatively affect your growth, and know what these things are, then all you have to do to positively affect your growth is slightly adjust some of those things according to what you will learn in this book.

As you probably noticed, the most shocking fact was shown in the study from Journal of Biosocial Science, that about 20% or even more of body height depends on person's environment (where and how you live). That is a big number! It means that a person can become over 20% taller than his parents is that person's environment is much better then what his parents had when they were young. It happens often these days. It also means that every person has at least some potential to become taller than what he destined to be without any additional actions.

Before we finally start learning what to do, let me give you few other reports that should completely remove any doubts from anyone who previously thought that height of a person cannot be affected by anything but genes.

According to a 2004 report in Economics and Human Biology, *"studies of escapees from North Korea show that those born after the partitioning of the Korean Peninsula in the North were consistently about two inches shorter than their counterparts in the South".*

In a study called "Height and weight differences between North and South Korea" by Daniel Schwekendiek, an economist from the University of Tuebingen in Germany, compared 2002 data that showed *"preschool children in North Korea were up to 5 inches (12.7 cm) shorter and up to 14 pounds (6 kg) lighter than children who were brought up in South Korea. A 2006 study of 1,075 North Korean defectors aged 20 to 39 put the difference for adults at 4 inches (10 cm) for men and 2.5 (6.4 cm) inches for women. The studies blame malnutrition in North Korea for the height difference".*

These height differences are stunning because before the Korea was divided during the World War II into North and South, all Koreans were more or less of the same size. Just because North Korea is a most isolated country in the world, where almost no people can get in or out, this unfortunate experiment took place. There is also an extreme difference between young North Koreans and older North Koreans who grew up before the country's economies became much worse in 1990s. **This experiment clearly showed us on a big scale how much can the same people become so much different physically just because of different environments and economies they live in**.

> *Starting in the mid 1990s, North Korean leader ordered people to do special exercises designed to make them taller, including hanging from rings or parallel bars for as long as 30 minutes. For the same reason Basketball recently became a national sport in North Korea.*

Another similar example was observed by the anthropologist Barry Bogin. When in the early 1970s when about a million of Mayan Indian men from Guatemala fled to the United States during the Guatemalan Civil War, he measured their adults' average height. By the year 2000, the average height of Guatemalan Maya who fled at young age, became about 4 inches (10 cm) taller. This clearly shows how better nutrition and lifestyle can affect height so significantly.

Another report from 2004: *The Vietnamese government is worried by studies that show its population is not growing taller as fast as the populations of countries like China and Japan. So the state-run Physical Training and Sports Institute has proposed a solution. Its $40 million program would set up diet and exercise standards at public schools to bolster children's height and weight. The goal is to add 3 centimeters to the height of kids by 2010.*

An interesting study was also shown by economic historian John Komlos and Benjamin Lauderdale in Social Science Quarterly: *Americans were "tallest people in the world between colonial times and the middle of the 20th century", have now "become shorter (and fatter) than Western and Northern Europeans. In fact, the U.S. population is currently at the bottom end of the height distribution in advanced industrial countries." Komlos and Lauderdale believe this might be explained by the fact that children in the U.S. eat more meals that are "prepared outside the home," which tend to be high in fat and low in nutrients.* The report includes factors like health, safety, diet and family relationships.

In a report issued by Unicef in 2007, showing measures of child well-being in 21 rich countries, including health and safety, family and peer relationships and such things as whether children eat fruit and are physically active. The report put the Netherlands at the top, so the Dutch are now the world's tallest people, almost 3 inches taller, on average, than non-Hispanic American whites. The U.S. ended up in 20th place, below Poland, Portugal and Hungary, but ahead of Britain. This shows us how lifestyle and diet of average American is changing, and as a result – changing average height.

As you can see from all these reports above, it is a well-known and documented fact that people's environment, activities and diet seriously affect people's height. You can also see that even governments recognize that exercise and diet can affect people's growth. *My studies and experiments for over many years had shown the same.* All this statistical information may not be in much interest to you, however ***it is crucial for you to understand and truly believe that your height is in your hands and it is in your power to change it.***

Remember *– our doubts are the main if not the only enemy we have. Thoughts like "what if it will not help?" or "the week past by, but where are the results?" are diminishing your efforts, often completely blocking any of your progress. It is wise to search for advise from people when you absolutely sure they know the correct answer. However, I strongly recommend not to ask for advise from sources you are not sure of having enough expertise. It is the rule with anything we are trying to accomplish in our lives, including gaining height. Asking the wrong person often not only gives no results or incorrect information, but seeding doubts in your ability to accomplish your desire. Doubts of a person are infectious to almost anyone who listens that person expressing those doubts. That is why it is often better to keep your desire away from people who may not believe in your results. In other words, just read this book, follow it, accomplish you what you desire, then spread the news on what you have accomplished if you want. You can tell your goals today only to your closest friends and those who you think would benefit from this book as well.*

The average person, no matter what height he or she is, has a potential to be taller by 2 – 5 inches. Why then most people are shorter than they could be? Simply, because they don't know how to make most of their potential or just don't believe that it could be done. Know that ***any victory depends not from circumstances that you face, but from how you view those circumstances.***

The Power of Thought

You may think – what our thoughts have to do with increasing height? **Everything!** What I'm about to explain will be the most crucial information in your quest to achieve your desire.

Yes, our thoughts have a lot of power and we can use this power to accomplish anything, including growing taller. This may not be easy to understand for many people because they may never heard of this, but I will try to explain and prove that this is true and very important. If you will not understand why, you will not accomplish much.

Everything in the Universe is created by thoughts. People and all other living creatures were created and shaped by thoughts. Yes, even the evolution is the direct result of thoughts living creatures had over millions of generations. I have been thinking about this for many years, and now it is in my true believe, even though this evolution theory has never been brought-up by anyone before. The way your body including your face looks right now is the direct result of all your thoughts you've had during the course of your entire life. You don't believe me? Can you tell a difference in appearance between a person that had been a homeless for many years and a successful wealthy person? What about a very smart and mentally challenged? Have you ever thought why people with Down syndrome often look alike? Because their thoughts are very basic and not strong enough for their faces to be changed. We all look different because we all think different. If people would loose their thinking abilities, they would all look like people with Down syndrome.

Look at people around you or on TV. Can you spot unsuccessful and very successful people not even knowing them? There are hundreds of clues, but I will mention just the simplest one to spot: you will never find a person who has been very successful and had fulfilled life for many years with a very small chin. You will also rarely find a person that has never had much success in his life with a very large chin. Why successful people have larger chins? The answer you will find in this simple experiment: try to imagine yourself as en extremely wealthy and successful person with unlimited powers, able to accomplish anything you want. Don't just think it could be you, truly think that you are that person, thinking, looking, and behaving like one. Hold that thought for a minute. Do you feel any difference? Try to recognize expression on your face, how it changes, how does your face feel? Do you feel any sensation inside your chin? Do you feel how your chin is trying to extend? I bet you do. It is a normal but unintentional reaction every person has when he or she has great self-confidence. If you hold that thought for much longer, believe it or not, your chin will start growing, among other changes of your face expression and in some ways – other parts of your body. *By the way, if you hold that thought long enough, you will become that person.* This is a **big secret of life,** the rule that you cannot escape – *you are who you think you are*. In other words, *you become what you think about the most*. Remember this for the rest of your life.

These examples show us that our thoughts do have power to change the shape of the body.

I will give you few other simple examples that show how our thoughts have direct affect on physical reality around us, including events that occur with us, and results that we are trying to accomplish. You may probably think that this is not our subject, just be patient and you will understand that it is.

When you throw a ball into a basket or any other object into a target, try to visualize the trajectory of the flying object and exact point where the object will have to end-up. You must clearly imagine that object at the point of your interest like it is already there, before you throw. As you practice, you will be amazed how much better you will be at that than before. Your thoughts will practically materialize.

Regardless of how old you are, I'm sure you've had bad periods and good periods in your life. Try to remember what triggered those periods to become bad or good. Do you remember some negative thoughts you've had before something bad happened to you? What about positive thoughts before you had accomplished something good? If you don't remember, ask other people. Many people don't realize it, but they create their own reality with their thoughts. Have you heard of expression: "Be careful what you wish for"?

Are you starting to understand why I am trying to explain to you all this? Right, **your mind has a lot of power to boost your body's growth rate, among many other things**. Only full understanding of your powers will give you those powers, so read on.

Did you know that you can actually heal yourself from almost any disease using your thoughts alone? All you have to do is to clearly visualize and feel your affected organ, then mentally remove the disease from this organ. You do need a good understanding of the disease, your organ's position and it's functions though. With good practice it can be done. As strange as this may sound, it is true, and there are many people who know this technique and use it. Next time when you have some pain anywhere in your body, concentrate your thought on the place where the pain is coming from, trying to relax that area as you would relax a muscle. You can also imagine your pain as some object that does not belong there, and try to remove it by your thought. If you take it seriously, you will be surprised how well this can work.

> _Can you think of anything that was ever made by people that was not created first in their heads? Our entire man-made reality was invented with our thoughts, and it will be correct to say that anything that we do was done at lease twice: first time with our thoughts, and then – with our hands._

Let me give you another important piece of information: There is now scientific evidence proving just how important our thoughts can be to health and personal well-being. Recent studies show that DNA can be influenced and reprogrammed by thoughts WITHOUT cutting out and replacing single genes. Think about it, **_even the main molecule that gives instructions to our body on how to develop can be changed by our thoughts!_**

Do you believe now that you can increase your height with your thoughts? Good, but just to believe is not enough. **Don't waste time; start doing it right now, while reading this.**

> **_Imagine your whole body beginning to stretch-out and grow, literally instructing your bones to grow._** _Do you feel anything? Practice and you should feel how body stretches and grows. Hold that thought for as long as you can concentrate. Congratulations, you have just given your body a very important and powerful assignment, and the body will do everything needed to fulfill that assignment._

Let me clarify a very important point. Our thoughts do materialize, but not all of them. Thoughts that appeared for a few seconds as a flash and disappear, as they never existed, don't have much power. The exception to this is when we have many small negative thoughts or many small positive thoughts within some period of time. Those can materialize into some negative or positive events. **_A thought has the real power when it is "alive" for a long time._** Please understand that your "hopes" are also not powerful thoughts. **_Powerful thoughts are exact mental instructions that take time to "cook" in order for them to materialize._**

Now, with the understanding of what our thoughts are capable of, it is important for you to understand how it actually happens. This knowledge will help you to achieve better results. It may not be a simple subject, but I will try to make it as simple as possible for you.

Our body and everything around us is made of energy. The energy has an unlimited range of frequencies. For example, sound that we hear, radio waves, infrared, visible light, ultraviolet, and others frequencies known to science are just a very small fraction of all existing ranges of energy in the universe. It means that what we can see, hear and touch is not everything that exists; in fact it's just an incredibly small fraction of energy waves compared to what we cannot see, hear or touch. Therefore, we can safely say that _our physical bodies consist of much more than what we can touch or see, even in microscope._

This will bring us to the following: there is a **substance or energy** of a higher frequency located exactly where the physical body is located, shaped exactly how the physical body is shaped, including all organs. We could think that this substance is just the energy that our body radiates, but it is exactly the opposite. The physical body with its shape and condition is just a lower frequency duplicate of that substance. In fact, **that substance is what we are**; our mind and soul are parts of that substance. If the physical body dies, the mind and its energy substance will live on. In fact, _the only reason for our physical existence is for our mind to experience life at lowest frequencies (which is our physical universe) and learn from it._ Yes, you live because you want to learn, and everything that is happening to you, including reading this book, is your mind's learning curve to progress itself into higher dimensions. Our mind can be compared to a computer's hard drive, and our brain is just a processor for the body to function properly. And yes, your mind may move into another body after your physical life is finished, as the hard drive can be moved to another computer.

Why am I giving you all this? Because you need that knowledge in order to understand the following: _our thoughts are the energy our mind produces._ What does it mean? It means – our energy substance and our thoughts are made of the same material, and our thoughts can directly affect and control our energy substance (let's call it "energy twin"). Ah-ha, does it mean that **if our thoughts can change the shape and size of our energy twin, our physical body will follow it**? You've got it right!

As you already know, our entire body and its every organ are made of trillions of tiny cells that can be seen only in powerful microscope. But did you know that **about 98% of the all the cells of your body are replaced by new cells every year**? *Yes, your skin, all organs and even your bones are being replaced constantly.*

This is how it works: our body take in new atoms from the air we breathe, the food we eat, and the liquids we drink. These atoms incorporate into our cells, replacing the old ones and fuel the chemical processes that keep us alive. The DNA molecule in each cell copies itself over and over again giving instructions on how these cells should be formed. These instructions are not exactly precise and slightly change according to the blueprint you hold in your subconscious or energy twin. Are you following? Above statement clearly explains how your thoughts and emotions do change the shape of your body inside and out.

You see, it was all worth it. Just keep in mind that you cannot turn yourself into some giant creature with seven legs and a tail just because you want to. There are limitations that were set in our genes and DNA that will not allow this to happen. It means **you have the power to increase the size of your body using your thoughts**, within a certain limit that we have discussed previously.

Growing Energy Twin

Armed with this new knowledge lets try again the exercise on instructing your body to grow. Stretch yourself and again imagine your whole body, your spine, and your legs stretching and growing. Try to feel the sensation of growing, at the same time visualizing your body already few inches taller. When you do that, your energy twin does actually get taller. It is not visible to untrained eyes, but there are people who have trained themselves to see people's aura, that could actually see your energy twin extended.

Now you know ***one of the most powerful secrets to reach your goal***. Do it as often as you can, holding that thought for as long as possible. This way eventually you will get used to that thought and sensation of growing to the extent of doing it as a habit. ***Your physical body will have no chance but to grow*** to fill-up the gap. Its like when you put a plant to grow in a little box, it's roots have only this much room to grow, but when you increase the size of the box – the plant's roots will eventually fill-up the extra space.

This visualization process will be an important part of almost all aspects in our quest to gain height. You will see references to this method of using the power of your thought throughout this book, and if you did not understand it fully, please read it over as many times as you need, to grasp the whole concept.

> As unbelievable as it may sound, what I gave you here are ***basic principals of life in the Universe***, this is how every living creature changes itself when surrounding environment forces to do that change to survive, *this is how evolution works*, and ***this is how you can change***. I am encouraging you to take these principals seriously because they not only can be used to increase your height, but for anything you would like to accomplish in your life. In fact, most very successful people in the world know about this secret knowledge about the power of thought, and use it wisely.

Well, using the thought technique is a great and powerful start, but you need to help your body to grow with **all** techniques at our disposal. This will bring us to the next important issue – the hormone naturally produced in our body that is more responsible for our body's growth than anything else. This hormone is called "Human Growth Hormone".

Human Growth Hormone

Let me first explain what hormones are and what makes them so special. Don't try to remember all this, as you don't need to, but do not skip it either. I just want you to have at least slight understanding of what we are talking about, and its importance.

Hormones are chemicals produced by special cells in glands and other organs of the body; most hormones are produced by cells in the endocrine glands. Hormones are produced in very small amounts and released into the bloodstream, traveling to the "target organ" or tissue where they exert their effect. Several hormones are involved in regulating growth. Some act directly on target organs, while others act by triggering the production of other hormones, which activate specific organ functions necessary for growth.

The hormone that involved the most in regulating tissue growth and repair is Human Growth Hormone (HGH), which is a protein, made of building blocks known as amino acids. Growth hormone is produced particularly by the pituitary gland. Located in the center of our brain, the pituitary gland is often called the master gland because it plays a central role in many of different physiologic events producing a wider array of hormones than any other gland in the body. Those hormones regulate a number of essential physiological functions, including water and energy balance, influencing sexual development, metabolism, female menstrual cycle, mineral and sugar content of the blood, reproductive activity and the work of many other glands in the body. It maintains the efficiency of the various structures and prevents the excessive accumulation of fats.

It is growth hormone however that plays a significant role in energy production, muscle and tissue growth, fat loss, brain function, metabolic development, healing capacity, and strengthening bones and joint cartilages. It means that as much as it is important for body's growth in young age, *high (but not pathological) natural levels of growth hormone in grown-ups also extremely important if they want a longer and healthier life.* For that purpose I strongly suggest grown-ups, who want to rebuild their body and keep it in shape, to read this book and follow along with their younger ones.

Our goal should be to increase the level of growth hormone released into your bloodstream, and there are many ways this can be done, naturally and unnaturally. I'm firmly suggesting only natural ways, but because many people are often seriously considering using different man-made products to boost their growth hormone level, we will briefly go over those with complications they may cause.

There are two unnatural ways to increase growth hormone level:

1)   Using ***growth hormone releasing products*** like glycine, glutamine, agrinine, ornithine, niacin, and 16 other amino acids you can get with or without prescription. These substances and drugs are usually used by bodybuilders. They are also useful for elderly people to increase their growth hormone level. Some of them are good for boosting immunity, protecting the liver, fighting cancer, helping rebuild body tissue after surgery or trauma, and there are many other applications. Because amino acids help produce growth hormone, some of them, with proper exercises, may actually trigger some positive effect on your growth. However, I would not recommend doing this self-treatment without medical supervision, especially for children. Any of these drugs has to be taken in proper dosage. Some of them need to be combined with other drugs or nutrients. Improper usage may cause you serious problems. And there are many side effects from using these products: diarrhea, low toxicity, headache, drowsiness, muscle spasms, dizziness, high blood pressure, nervousness, depression, hair loss, gaining weight, and many more. So, be careful.

2)   ***Man-made growth hormone*** is administered by a series of injections or orally (which could cost anywhere from $12,000 to $26,000 a year in young children and can exceed $50,000 a year in adolescents), and is prescribed after careful evaluation of a person's growth pattern and growth potential. These injections may help you grow, but inducing growth too quickly may inhibit later growth. Possible side effects of man-made growth hormone injections are very extensive: high cholesterol, diabetes, liver abnormalities, increased tissue stiffness, carpal tunnel syndrome, musculoskeletal disease, neuropathy, allergic reactions, pancreatitis, hyperglycemia, visual deterioration, headaches, vomiting, increased liver enzyme levels, increased sweating, edema, ear infection, abdominal pain or bloating, changes in vision, pain in general and back pain specifically, nausea and vomiting, skin rash or itching, carpal tunnel syndrome, enlargement of breasts, muscle pain, fatigue and swelling of hands. Injecting growth hormone causes muscles to grow bigger but mushy and weak and joints to become painful… Should I give you more or is it enough for you to think at least twice before you go that direction?

> if you receive man-made growth hormone injections, your body will adapt to this drug, and will refuse to produce natural growth hormone after you stop receiving injections.

I hope you have made the right choice, and if the choice is to artificially increase HGH level, I'm once again strongly suggest to consult a good doctor. If you think these procedures are not for you, read further…

There are **numbers of ways to stimulate the increase of growth hormone release in your body naturally.** Those include ***resistance or high-intensity exercise, dieting strategies, enough sleep, fasting, stimulating reflex zones,*** even ***state of your awareness and mood.*** Lets discuss all of them in detail:

Resistance or high-intensity exercise

Resistance or high-intensity exercise is *the most powerful way to increase growth hormone level*. As part of this program, you will need to do different types of exercises, and resistance or high-intensity exercises will be shown as part of the exercise program, all of which will be show in the later chapter. It is scientifically proven that pituitary gland releases of growth hormone can be triggered by a physical stress during a *relatively short* period of time and by exercise-induced increases in adrenaline. It means that regular low-intensity exercise may be somewhat good for regular growth hormone increase, but even few seconds of pushing yourself closer to the limit releases more growth hormones than days of slow-pace exercises. Please don't get me wrong, slow-pace exercises are very important; in fact most exercises in this program are slow-pace.

There are many types of exercise you can perform that may include high-intensity periods. Those could be cycling, swimming, skiing, weight lifting (read "weight lifting" section of this book before you do this), push-ups, running, or even power walking. It can be performed in the gym on an elliptical trainer, stationary bike, recumbent bike, or a treadmill.

There was a study performed by researchers from University of North Carolina and University of Virginia with maximal cycle ergometer exercise at different pedaling rates, comparing cyclist's growth hormone levels when they were resting after a 6 second cycle sprint, and after 30 second cycle sprint at maximum speed. Researchers also measured growth hormone level afterwards to see how long HGH stayed in participant's bodies after exercise. The results were incredible: The 6 second sprint method did move growth hormone level a little, but the 30 second of full effort sprint experiment increased growth hormone level by 5 times over resting baseline and 4 times over the lesser intensity sprint. According to the researchers, growth hormone level stayed elevated for 1.5 to 2 hours after the sprinting program. Another important finding was showing that if a cyclist repeated full-

effort sprint shortly after the first sprint, the level of growth hormone did not show any additional increase. Moreover, the growth hormone released during exercise also targets body fat for up to two hours after training, so those who are thinking to lose weight should also take a notice on this.

Based on all of the above and my own research, I would recommend to perform resistance or high-intensity exercise daily, or at least three times per week. It is also *very important not to over-do it*. **Do it no more then 3 times per day with at least 2.5 hours in between**. Also, you cannot do it unprepared. You have to prepare your body by performing the same or different exercise that involves the same muscles in a much slower, relaxed pace for at least several minutes before pushing to the limit. **Pushing to the limit should be somewhere between 20 and 60 seconds, and stopping should be gradual, not very fast**. If you feel that you cannot hold it any longer, gradually stop high-intensity but continue to move the same muscles in a much-relaxed mode for at least a minute.

High-intensity exercise, if it is done properly, is very good for general health, for the cardiovascular system, and especially for strength training. However, my goal is not to teach you how to get stronger, but to show you how to grow taller, while making you healthier and more successful in anything that you do. That is why I will stress-out once again not to over-do your high-intensity exercise; moreover, if you have any concerns over your health, please consult a doctor before performing any stressful physical activity.

Enough sleep

Getting enough sleep is also one of the most important factors in increasing growth hormone level. It is a well-known fact that the largest portion of growth hormone is released during sleep. And it does not occur immediately as we go to sleep, but mostly during the deep level sleep, which usually starts after about 90 minutes of sleep. In fact, scientists observed that about 70% of growth hormone release occurring during the sleep is associated with slow-wave sleep or deep level sleep. You will learn everything you need to know on this issue in a later chapter about sleep, and I'm advising you to read that as a very important piece of information.

Dieting strategies

Dieting strategies will be explained in great detail later in this book, but I will give you several major factors that affect the release of growth hormone which you need to understand now because they are crucial.

Before I do that, I want you to realize how actually important *what to eat and how*. The expression "you are – what you eat" is not far from the reality (we are discussing the body in this case, not the soul), even though sometimes you may think you look healthier and stronger eating junk food than your friend that eats only healthy food. If you think that way, wait for another 20 years and look at your friend and yourself. I can guarantee – you will be very surprised and will understand that "you are – what you eat" statement is true, the hard way.

You may not be thinking too much about your future 20 or more years from now, but if you will eat poorly and unhealthy today, these are the facts you will have to face later, regardless of what you think: *you will be shorter than could be; you will live at least several years less than you could, possibly even several decades less; as you will age, you may suffer from many painful diseases; you may be well overweighed; your memory may diminish sooner than you think; you will feel powerless, unhappy, and your looks will not be attractive.* You don't believe me? Ask a bad looking unhealthy person in his or her 50th or 60th how and what that person ate all his or her life, and ask a good looking healthy person of the same age the same question. You create your future now, and eating right is a very big part of creating the better future.

Growth hormone production depends very much on the level of carbohydrates in food that we eat and the amount of insulin that those carbohydrates help to produce. In addition, some foods contain *amino acids* that are favorable to the production of growth hormone, as well as *fat*, the correct balance of which should be kept at all times for maximum results. Growth hormone production is also dependent upon *adequate levels of Zinc, Magnesium and Potassium. Timing of food intake* plays an important role as well. We will discuss all of that in full detail later.

Just so you know, several scientific groups have concluded that *obesity does reduce the production of growth hormone.* That should be another reason for you to eat right and exercise.

> *Don't be discouraged simply because it all may look little too complicated for you. All this is actually not complicated at all if you read it carefully. Just study food intake suggestions in full detail later in the book and you will be just fine following those suggestions.*

Fasting

Fasting for at least 24 hours can also give a good signal to a pituitary gland to produce more of a growth hormone. It is a very good practice to fast for a full day at least once a month or even better – every 2 weeks because health benefits can be enormous, but what may be even more important for you is that it helps to increase the release of growth hormone.

Fasting allows the insides of your body to take a bath, cleansing itself from all its toxins. However, I will not promote fasting as an absolutely necessary part of this program. If you will still decide to do this, I would recommend that you ask your physician if fasting is safe for your health. Some health problems might not allow you to fast.

For most people, not eating for 24 hours is not an easy task, especially in the beginning. You should prepare yourself for two days before fasting by switching to a light diet. Salads, juices, and cooked vegetables should be your preference on these days. Meat, fish, dairy products, and breads should be avoided. As you get closer to the fasting day, you should eat less and less, so that you keep yourself a little hungry.

For fasting, you should choose a day when you are not so busy. During fasting you should drink a lot of water (will be discussed in detail later in the book), and at times when you usually have breakfast, lunch and diner, you can drink vegetable or/and fruit juices. 3 to 4 hours before going to sleep is usually the best time to have the last meal, having the next light meal on the next day also 3 to 4 hours before going to sleep.

Stimulating Reflex Zones

Every part and every organ of our body is connected with at least several areas somewhere on the body's surface, and is affected if these areas are stimulated. This rule applies to the pituitary gland as well. It means that there are certain areas on the body that positively affect the work of the pituitary gland if stimulated, which directly affects the increased release of growth hormone into the body. These areas are called **reflex zones**.

One such zone is located on a **small area near the center of the pad of the each big toe** (called **pituitary gland reflex point**). To find this point, imagine a line drawn down the center of a big toe and another line crossing it horizontally at the widest points of the big toe. The pituitary gland reflex area is where these lines cross. Another effective way to find the exact location of the pituitary reflex point on your own feet is using the eraser-end of a pencil and firmly, yet gently, begin pressing into the center of your big toes. Gradually move the eraser slightly to the right and then the left of the point, as you continue pressing – you will eventually find the point where it hurts – that's where the zone is. To stimulate that spot, simply place the big toe between your thumb and index finger. Apply pressure and press in an upward motion. Repeat the process on the opposite foot. You can do it with eraser-end of a pencil as well by continuing a constant pressure with the point for approximately 1 minute – then release the pressure. Repeat 3 times.

Another great way to stimulate this reflex point is by walking, walking on your toes, running and especially jumping (will be described in detail in the exercise program of this book). *Barefooted is preferred.*

An important suggestion: drink at least a glass of water before you massage your foot.

Another such zone is located at the **point near the center of the pad of the each thumb.** It is often located off center; it can be slightly higher, lower, to the right or to the left. With your other hand place the thumb in between your other hand's thumb and index finger. Apply pressure to the middle of the tip of the thumb directly behind the fingernail then press around until you find a point where it slightly hurts. This is a pituitary gland zone. To stimulate, apply pressure in an upward motion repeatedly for 1 minute on each thumb. Repeat 3 times.

The final reflex zone that stimulates the pituitary gland is the **hollow spot between your eyebrows where your forehead and nose meet.** To stimulate it, keep your eyes closed as you apply pressure to this point for about two minutes. You can lie down while pressing this point as well.

There is also another powerful way to stimulate this point – **mental focus:** Sit down comfortably on the chair leaning back. Bring your head all the way back. Begin breathing deeply while focusing on the point in between your eyebrows. Imaging the air coming in and out of that point as you breath-in and breath-out accordingly. Continue for one minute.

Because the pituitary gland not only affects your body's development, but also harmonizes any imbalance within the body, stimulating it with procedures shown above will effectively relax and energize you. That is why these are great ways to reenergize yourself after exercise or any other time when you are tired.

It also great if done right before bedtime – to help calm and relax your body, as well as right after you wake-up in the morning – to help naturally "jump-start" your energy level.

Later in this book you will learn about performing self-massage to stimulate your body's development. It is best to combine stimulation of reflex zones with massage.

State of your awareness and mood

State of your awareness and mood, surprisingly, is also a powerful factor when it comes to the production of growth hormone in our bodies, and it had been scientifically proven.

> *Several studies that compared normal children and children with depression had shown severe negative effect on growth hormone secretion in psychologically depressed children. The development of human body and its condition very much depends on our average mood.*

Every organ and process in our body reacts to our thoughts (read "Power Of Thought" chapter of this book) and our current state of mind. If you feel distressed for a long time for example, whatever the reason is, your whole body will react accordingly slowing down every development process, including the release of human growth hormone. On the opposite, feeling good about yourself and everything around you, thinking only positive will definitely have a positive effect on all processes in your body, especially growth hormone release. Remember – *your physical body and your mind are made of the same substance – energy, just of different frequencies (and dimensions), which are directly connected as a whole.*

I'm sure you feel positive about great results you are about to accomplish and about your bright and healthy future! If so, your energy twin and your physical body are at full speed working to help you achieve just that, growth hormone is releasing in more quantities as you read this right now. Your thoughts are materializing!

What if I don't feel so positive, you would ask? Well, it's easy to fix. How about making a smile right now? Yes, while you are reading these words. Just do it even if you don't want to, at least for 10 seconds. Do you feel anything different? If you are still alive, you should feel your mood improving almost constantly, your positive thoughts are coming back to you, you just feel better. It is a normal reaction that shows us how easy it is to change the state of our awareness in any situation. You see, *a simple smile can increase the release of growth hormone into your body.* Do you want to feel even better? Easy. Just think of anything that makes you really happy. It could be an object, a place, an event, a person, something from your past or something imaginary. It really makes no difference what it is or who it is, as long as you can clearly visualize it and it reminds you of true happiness. Let's say you've spent the best moments of your childhood on a beautiful sandy beach. Try to remember and visualize this place as clear as possible, imagine yourself there right now, as if a time machine brought you back there. If you do that and it will not improve you mood, nothing will.

If you want real results, smile and say to yourself: "I'm on my way to success". Remember – ***your thoughts do materialize.***

If you have read all of the above, I am congratulating you on learning *the most valuable information you could have on how the growth process works and what has to be done to improve it.* If you did not read it yet or did not fully understand the importance of all this material, please read it. It is crucial to understand the basics before we move-on to other activities that follow in this program, which are also very important part of your quest to reap maximum benefits from this book.

Water

I want to stress-out the importance of this chapter. Please do not skip it and take what I write seriously. You may follow everything what I recommend in this book, but without following this chapter you will unlikely see any significant results.

> Did you know that about three out of four parts of our body consist of water? Yes, we are largely made of water and fully depend on it. Water is involved in almost every biological process in our body. It regulates body's temperature, moisturizes skin, maintains muscle strength, and lubricates all joints. Water is essential to form good blood, skin, healthy tissues, and it gives us the energy of life. We cannot survive even a few days without water.

You may probably heard from your doctor to drink more water, most doctors do recommend that, but you may never hear from them that most diseases are actually caused by luck of plain water in your body. Yes, most of diseases humans suffer are simply varieties of thirst. The official modern medicine claims that thirst is when you feel dryness in your mouth with subconscious thought of wanting to drink. This is *one of major mistakes of modern medicine* because most people become thirsty only as the last stage of thirst – when most of the water is sucked out of all organs. This is what damages those organs, forcing people to run to doctors who are trying to cure us with drugs that damage organs even more. Instead, all we have to do is just drink enough water for our organism to function properly.

The reason why we have no thirst even when our body badly needs it is the ability of our body to adapt to most difficulties it may encounter.

When you are drinking less and less water, the brain recognizes the luck of water and adapting to the situation, putting the body in the surviving mode. The brain gives the signal to increase the release of special neurotransmitter – *histamine* that is responsible for distributing water throughout the body. Histamine starts prioritizing where to store the water that left in the body, giving most of the water to organs that need it most for the body to survive, at the same time working as temporary water substitute releasing energy for the body to function and diminishes the pain the dehydration causes.

This reflex was inherited from our ancestors over millions of years in order to survive when they really had no access to enough water for long periods of time. If we wouldn't have that reflex, we would die from thirst even with slight dehydration.

As you probably figured out already, your body's growth depends on proper functioning of all your organs, which depend on proper water balance in your body. **If you want to grow, make sure you drink enough water.**

The importance of water in our road to success is so great, that I want to give you some facts that you need to know to understand this importance before I will explain you how to drink and what to drink (which is also crucial).

This water that we take for granted as something very simple and basic is actually so much more complex than most of us can ever imagine. In order for you to really appreciate it, lets briefly look at the history of water and some of its abilities.

Did you know that the water that you drink today is the same water that dinosaurs drank over 160 million years ago, as well as first alive organisms that appeared on earth billions of years ago? Water is one of the main ingredients for life to exist in this three dimensional universe. It exists on countless planets throughout universe, in fact – space is virtually littered with unimaginable amounts of frozen water, which falls in hundreds of thousands of tons on planets in its path every day, including Earth. If the planet is too hot – the water simply vaporize and don't reach the surface of that planet; if the planet is too cold – the ice simply builds on its surface; if the planet is just worm as our Earth – that intergalactic ice falls into the planet's atmosphere turning into clouds as it heats-up by the collision, eventually falling as water on the planet's surface as it cools-off. What it all means is that most of the water on our planet actually came from space, accumulating over billions of years. Moreover, life itself came from the space with that water, started in the water, flourishing and evolving into millions of different organisms, some of which came out of water but still fully depended on it. Environment was changing over millions of years, and with environment all living creatures in order to survive were changing too, slowly turning into all organisms that live today, including people. As you can see, we all not only depend on water, we came from water and *we are water*, for the most part.

This simple water is probably the most complex substance in the Universe. Its abilities are endless and scientists are just starting to comprehend the power of water.

This is not a science book, but some things that I believe are too important to miss I prefer to explain in little more detail, so you could understand why it is so important. *Understanding and believing is much more powerful than just believing, and it is much easier to believe in something when you have more-or-less full understanding of what you believe in.* As you've probably noticed, I'm trying my best to explain everything in simplified manner because I'm writing it for you, my young feller – not for a scientific community. Therefore, don't miss anything, it's important.

Water as a substance has chemical and physical properties like no other substance, in its liquid state, solid state (ice), and gaseous state (water vapor or steam). We will not get into much detail on this. I will just mention some things the water can do:

◆ Water is the main dissolvent for all food that we eat with its vitamins and minerals, making it possible for the food to be digested, transporting all the nutrients throughout the body.

◆ Water is the main source and regulator of energy in our body.

◆ Water gives the food that we eat necessary energy, and without water food cannot release its energy.

◆ The DNA molecule that controls our body's structure very much dependent on the presence of water. Within a living cell, each molecule of protein is surrounded by thousands of molecules of water. DNA – the essential protein for life – is held together by a hydrogen bond, the same one that holds the water around it. That means we can't look at DNA as a free-standing molecule; it is an integral part of a huge water cluster. The communication between these clusters is what makes physical life possible. *Absence or lack of water seriously damages the DNA, its reproduction process and its repair system affecting the body's development and growth*, also speeding-up the aging process.

◆ Water is absolutely necessary for the production of all hormones in the body. ***Increase of water consumption increases the release of growth hormone*** by the pituitary gland in the brain, also improving the distribution of hormones throughout the body.

◆ Every one of trillions of cells in our body fights for water, and when there is not enough water in the body – less important cells simply die out.

◆ Water actually keeps the structure of each cell intact.

◆ Water is the ***main lubricate*** in all growth plates in bones and spine disks making it possible for plates to be stimulated at their maximum, which increases body's growth.

- The cartilage in the body, including all joints, is composed mainly of water, luck of which will decrease the ability of the cartilage to repair itself.

- The brain is the most "water hungry" organ in the body, and it functions with much better efficiency with increase of water consumption. If you want to increase the brainpower – drink up.

- Drinking more water releases stress and depression.

- As you already know, the most growth hormone is released during the deep sleep at night. Enough water in the body improves the quality of sleep and increases the time of deep level sleep. This is crucially important!

- Water increases the effectiveness of immune system, fighting any diseases that may affect your growth.

- *Increasing water intake is better than any diet for a person who wants to lose weight.* Almost always thirst is mistaken as hunger, so the person eats much more to remove that unpleasant feeling of, as he thinks, hunger. That feeling, more often than not, can be removed by drinking plain water. In dehydrated body, cells release their stored energy and starting to depend more on the energy that comes from food, increasing the fat production for the body to survive. Don't forget: *increasing weight may decrease your chance to grow taller*, so the water is your friend even here.

There is so much more I could say about water's powers, but I hope above said is more than enough for you to understand its importance. However, there is one more ability which water possesses that is not less important than of all of the above mentioned combined. It is the ability of water to absorb, carry and release information. Let me explain:

Everything in the Universe is energy and its variations. Every atom of every physical substance carries energy. This energy is actually a vibration of certain frequency. That vibration of atoms has its own static structure or a combination, which releases the energy. That energy is **information**. What it means is that every subject or substance carries information in the form of its own vibrational structure or model, radiating its energy into surroundings. What is even more interesting, that vibrational structure can change to a certain extent because not only it radiates its energy, but also absorbs informational energy from its surroundings as a sponge.

Yes, every stone or any other object or substance is "sensitive" to informational energies surrounding it, and can "influence" informational energies of objects and living creatures that are in contact with it. The level of sensitivity and energy exchange depends on the molecular structure of each material, which means those different stones or other materials have different abilities to store and release information.

Out of all materials and substances, *only water* stands-out as the most sensitive to its surrounding energies, and the best substance to "memorize" and share information it had acquired with its surroundings. It is so sensitive that it actually changes its properties depending on what type of energy it holds. Water from different sources will affect living organism differently if those sources had different surroundings. For example, spring water and tap water are different not only in how clean they are, but also in informational energy they possess. Spring water that never touched any plumbing usually has the purest energy that is most beneficial for our bodies. Tap water in cities usually goes from the reservoir through several filtration processes before it is pronounced fit for human consumption, then it goes through miles of piping until it gets to you. It not only has deposits of different particles from piping system, and missing important minerals that are found in spring water, but also lost all the pure energy it once had. Moreover, this water got the energy of piping and filtration systems.

Did you know that out of trillions of snowflakes you see fallen there will never be two flakes that look exactly the same? Why do you think is that? Because the shape of water crystals depends strictly on its current surrounding energies, and each water drop crystallizes as it falls into freezing air in its very unique point in space with its very unique energy frequency.

All of this brings us to the *main conclusion* – since water can "feel" the energy, and as we discussed earlier, our thoughts are the energy our mind produces, **the water feels our thoughts**. Not only it feels and absorbs our thoughts, **water's powers and abilities are also changing by our thoughts**. That is why I gave you lots of information above that could seem irrelative to the topic of this book; I hope you now understand why it is important.

The water that you drink will change its properties depending on your thoughts, your mood and even on what you think of that water. Therefore, it will affect your body differently depending on your thoughts and mood. If you drink water and thinking how terrible it is, don't even dream of getting any positive effects from this water, moreover – it can actually harm you. Even if you simply don't care about water's powers or don't believe in it, the water will not care about you either even if you drink lots of it. It may sound bizarre to you, but it is true.

> **Water is a living substance that can harm you or cure you, depending what energies it had been in contact with in the past and what energies you radiate when you are in contact with it.**

When drinking water, think of many positive things the water will help you with. Think how it will help you grow taller, how it will treat any disease that you have, how it will improve your brain function and your health in general.

I would advise you to checkout pictures of water crystals made by Masaru Emoto who became famous throughout the world because of those images. Just type his name in any search engine to find them. He made those pictures when freezing droplets of water starts to crystallize while giving water certain thought, feeling, saying or writing a word or a phrase. He often charged the water with certain energy by attaching piece of paper on which he wrote the word or a phrase (the energy of thought is always transformed into paper on which you write that thought). Remarkably, water reacted clearly showing what it likes or dislikes creating crystals strictly according to the message it had received. The most perfect and beautiful crystals were created after it received words "love", "friendship", and "thank you"; after receiving any negative messages, crystals formed shapes that were disproportionate and unpleasant to watch. If messages were too disturbing, crystals could not be formed at all. Mr. Emoto also took pictures of water crystals from many different sources and different conditions around the planet. Water from pristine mountain streams and springs always has beautifully formed geometric designs in their crystalline patterns. Polluted and toxic water from industrial and populated areas and stagnated water from water pipes and storage dams show definitively distorted and randomly formed crystals.

All this proves to us *not only that the water is a living and sensitive substance, but that our thoughts have real power and energy to affect anything they are pointed to, and they do materialize.*

Now, in light of all of the above, remember that our body consists mainly of water? Yes, that water that you are made of also reacts incredibly to your thoughts and feelings. Think about that, *since water is the main engine of all your body's functions and development, your thoughts and feelings do affect your body, its physical shape and condition.* Therefore, **your thoughts and feelings do affect your body growth**.

Have you noticed that people who think good of themselves, who try their best to stay positive and enjoying their lives are generally much healthier than those who think negatively of themselves, who often depressed, argue everything and rarely enjoy anything? Yes, it is always like that, thanks to water. *Next time when you feel negative about yourself, remember that you harm yourself that way on many different levels including your physical state.*

If you want to be healthier and grow taller, you have to love yourself, even if it may sound strange to you. And it is not shameful because if you cannot learn to love yourself, you cannot learn to love others. Remember, people will respect you much more if you will respect yourself. Also, based on what we've just learned, you should understand that your negative thoughts toward another person could harm that person's health as well, so be careful. If you do harm to others, harm will definitely by done to you in return sooner or later, that is *the law of life*. On the opposite, your good will and positive thinking about others will make their life better even if you didn't do anything physically and they don't even know about your thoughts. Sooner or later those good wills will return to you. Ask anyone much older than you are, and you will get the same answer.

If you want to grow taller, think positive, don't let your negative thoughts overwhelm you, think how water that is part of you and water that you drink working vigorously to increase your height. Before you drink water, think how good it is, feel your sincere gratefulness and love towards it for the life it gives you, for the health it gives you now and many years from now. If you do that, you will drink not just water; this water will change its properties and will become a true miracle drink that can cure anything and really help you to grow taller.

On a side note, sometimes it is not a good idea to tell your peers that you are "talking" to the water. Without knowledge that is given in this book, they might think – you are out of your mind. You will be much better off telling them to read this book first.

What to drink

First of all, when I mention water, I mean – *real plain water,* not any other liquid that contains water. All of these abilities and powers described above belong to water in its natural state only, without anything mixed into it. Yes, when the water is mixed with anything it changes its qualities. It does not mean those qualities are bad, but they will never be as good as in plain water regardless of what you will mix-in.

You may think that if you drink something that contains mostly water and satisfy your thirst should be good enough, but this would be misleading. Not only has the water lost best of its properties in most drinks we take, but also many drinks that were artificially produced contain particles that are damaging to our bodies. ***If you want to see great results from following my advises in this book,*** *I would strongly advise on quitting drinking any types of sodas, any drinks that have artificially created ingredients and anything that contain caffeine.*

Caffeine has one negative property among other things that will damage any of your efforts to increase the water level in your body. Caffeine triggers the reaction in the body to excrete more water through urination, rather than retaining it, dangerously dehydrating every organ. Even if you drink a lot of water, but often together with caffeine drinks, the water that you drink will not stay in the body, flashing out more than you take in. Caffeine drinks include coffee, tea, most soft drinks, and especially energy drinks. An exception to this would be teas that were lightly processed, containing low caffeine level such us green tea and especially white tea. White tea is made of only youngest tea buds collected from tea bushes, with a minimal amount of processing. It is one of the richest sources of antioxidants found in nature, and has considerably less caffeine than any other varieties of teas. A good quality white tea that is brewed correctly can give numerous health benefits at any age, but in no way it is better than plain pure water.

If you would have only two choices – to drink not so clean water as long as it has no dangerous bacteria or to drink manufactured drink, I would still recommend plain not so clean water. Nevertheless, water quality is extremely important.

The best water to consume is water that is clean from chemicals and bacteria, has some minerals that are important for health and energetically pure or clean from any negative energy. **The best drinkable water found in nature is spring water that was exposed to sunlight at least for a short while and was flowing with numerous curves.** When the water spins, it recharges its energy to the purest possible state, and while flowing through earth's deposits it mixes-in various important minerals.

The quality of tap water definitely varies in different towns and countries and generally not recommended to drink as-is, because as mentioned above, the water goes through various distribution systems, high pressure, chemical treatments and pipes, and can be contaminated with bacteria, pesticides, heavy metals, nitrates from fertilizers, and chlorine. Shockingly, more than 350 synthetic chemicals have been detected in some samples of tap water. The level of water contamination varies depending on where you live, but a certain number of chemicals are found across the board. That is why I would recommend having a tap water filtration or purification system at home. Also, regardless of how good your water filter is, it will never remove any negative energy from the water; moreover it may even add some of its own energy.

Let me share with you about one of the best ways to clean and reenergize tap water almost to the quality of fresh spring water. It is to *partially freeze the water, drain leftover dirty water and melt the clean ice.*

Just follow these steps:

1. *Put a bowl full of tap water into a freezer. The shape of the bowl should preferably be rounded, widening towards the top because if water will fully freeze, the ice will expand with the tremendous force and will break any container that has vertical walls. In the widening towards the top container, the ice will be pushed upwards.*

2. *Take it out from the freezer when about 1/2 – 2/3 of water is frozen. You will see one large bubble filled with water under relatively thin layer of ice. The time it takes to freeze depends on the temperature in your freezer and the size of the container; you just have to experiment to figure it out. I usually leave my 1.5 gallon bowls overnight.*

3. *Punch a hole with a knife right at the center or where the ice is thinnest and drain out all the water from the bubble. This water is dirty, and cannot be used.*

4. *Leave the ice in the container to melt for 30 – 45 minutes, and then drain out all melted water. It is done because there is some dirty water remaining on the outside layer of ice, so this step removes this dirt completely.*

5. *Leave the remaining ice to melt.*

This melted water is now purer than any water cleaned by filters. What happens here is that while the water crystallizes, it rejects all particles contained in it pushing them out. Slowly all dirty particles in the water concentrate in the middle while clean ice builds-up outside, creating a bubble of dirty water. If that dirty water is not flashed-out, it will freeze the last. If the water had a lot of particles in it, you would be able to see all this dirt concentrated in the middle.

If the water you are about to purify is very dirty, I still suggest filtering it first even with least expensive filter. Don't forget to change filters as often as suggested by their manufacturer. Often a coffee filter may be good enough for initial filtering.

The water that you will get this way is great for drinking, but to make the vibrational structure of water as close as possible to its original state, we should give that melted water a little spin. As unbelievable as it may sound, the water does regenerate itself when it goes through spinning movements as it does in nature when it flows between lots of stones.

One simple way to do it is just slowly pouring the water from one container to another, back and forth 5 – 10 times. The better way to do it is to connect two large soda bottles at their noses with one bottle full of water, then turn them up-side-down where the bottle with water is on top, slightly giving it a spinning motion. The water will flow down into an empty bottle in the spinning motion. The best way to connect these bottles is to use "tornado tube", which is a toy made for science experiments. It is very inexpensive ($2 – $3), just go to www.grow-taller.com/water where you will find a link to where it is sold.

As you do all this, don't forget to think of that water with full respect and thankfulness for all it gives you. Your thoughts will be "felt" by water, and it will respond with its increased powers.

You may think that all this is too time consuming. Yes, this process does take a long time, often a full day for the entire process (depending on amount of water in a bowl). However, all this will not take more than a total of 5 minutes of your time each day. To produce more clean water this way, have at least two water containers – while water melts in one, the other is in the freezer.

If you follow these techniques, you will create *the most powerful treatment your body could ever have*. This will be truly living water that will do wonders for your body's development and your health. This water can do many wonders, including helping anyone with any disease to recover faster, washing with it can make a skin healthier, even the hair can re-grow on bold people. If you will use this water for plants, as an example, you will see how much better they will grow;

even plants that could never survive in a low-light room will likely do very well there with this water. Therefore, if plants can grow better with good water, why can't you?

A simple way to check the quality of water is with the following experiment: *put one drop of water on a very clean flat piece of glass. You can tell the quality of the water by the shape of that drop. If the shape of a drop is spread and uneven, then the water is not pure and its vibrational structure is distorted. If the water is physically and structurally pure, as well as energized, the drop on the glass will look like a perfect pearl forming an almost perfect circle. The water purified by freezing and melting described above will pass this test.*

Another way of telling if you are drinking water that your body needs is by feeling it in your stomach. When you finish one of two glasses of water, you can feel right away if your body likes this water or not. Just slightly jump couple of times or just shake your body, and try to feel the water shaking in your stomach. If the water quality is very good and you body likes it, the water will be absorbed almost simultaneously as you drink it and you will simply not be able to feel a liquid in the stomach. If the water is not good enough, it will take much longer time to be absorbed, so you will feel the liquid shaking in the stomach.

Few words regarding plain water available for sale in bottles: Generally speaking, most bottled water is about the same quality as the tap water you would filter with an inexpensive filter because that is how this water is prepared. If the water called "spring water", it was not necessarily taken directly from the spring, more often then not – it's just filtered tap water, sometimes not even filtered.

Another factor affecting bottled water is – in what type of material the bottle is made of. As you know, most water bottles are made of plastic. That plastic is the most toxic plastic around – plastic number one. Lift any plastic water bottle and look underneath, and there you'll see a small triangle with the figure '1' inside it. This plastic is particularly toxic because over time it leaches chemicals and bacteria into the water, some of wich, such as substance called xenoestrogen, even negatively affect some hormones in the body. Bottles with the figure '2' or '3' inside the triangle are of much better quality, but the best quality you can get is in glass bottles.

When you buy the bottled water, check fine print on the labels. Only buy those brands that have very low sodium and calcium levels and a high magnesium content. Also, check the use-by date, and try to buy water that is as fresh as possible. And finally, don't buy carbonated mineral water because it deposits a lot of unwelcome gas in the stomach.

The best way for you to store your clean water is in glass containers. Even better – if you will also expose it to direct sunlight (you will understand why, as we will discuss this later in the book). Stainless steel or porcelain enamel finish containers are also fine to store the water.

How to calculate your daily water intake:

In US measurements: the *number of ounces* you should drink is *your body's weight in pounds divided by half.* For example, a 100-pound person should drink 100 / 2 = 50 oz of water. For reference, 1 cup of water is 8 oz. In this case 50 oz = 50 / 8 = approximately 6 caps of water.

In metric measurements: The *number of liters* you should drink is *your body's weight in kilograms divided by 32.* For example, a 45-kilogram person should drink 45 / 32 = 1.4 liters of water. For reference, 1 cup of water is 1/4 of one liter. In this case 1.4 liters = 1.4 X 4 = approximately 6 caps of water.

If you are involved with a lot of physical activities or live in a hot environment, the water intake should be 20% – 40% greater.

Fresh fruits and vegetables consist mostly of water (the best possible water you can have), also account into daily water intake. It means – you should decrease the amount of water you should drink by the amount of consumed fresh fruits or vegetables.

> A good way to tell if you are drinking enough water is the color of your urine. It should be either clear or very light. If the color is darker, you should increase your water intake.

You may think the amount of water you should drink is too much and not easy to handle. It well may be if you are not used to drinking water, but after a while (usually couple of weeks) your body will adapt to this and you will want to drink this much.

It is also extremely important how and when to drink water. These are the main rules:

◆ Drink 1 – 2 caps of water right before you go to sleep at night. This will give you better night sleep and will boost the release of the growth hormone.

◆ Drink 1 – 2 cups of water in the morning right after you wake-up to restore the loss of water during the night. Never miss a glass of water as you are getting up from the bed, and I can guarantee – you will add at least several years to your life. If you have breakfast without prior drinking a glass of water, you are doing a lot of damage to your body. You may also take one tablespoon of a good quality honey while drinking this first glass of water in the morning. Drink 2/3 of the water, eat honey, and then finish your water. This "morning start" will not only wake you up but also give you enough energy for morning exercises, even without breakfast.

◆ Drink 1 – 2 cups of water 30 minutes before meals. If you forgot to do that, it is still better to drink a cup of water even right before the meal than to skip it.

◆ Drinking during eating solid foods is not necessary (if you had a cup of water before the meal), but if you feel the need for water – you should definitely do it.

◆ You should not drink any water immediately and for 2 – 2½ hours after a meal. You have to let the food to digest, and the food is best digested if it falls into the water in the stomach, not when the water falls on top of food.

◆ The rest of the time, you should constantly drink water but in small amounts – few sips every 10 – 15 minutes. It is also a good practice to hold water in your mouth for a few seconds with every sip, moving it around in order to touch every surface inside the mouth before swallowing.

Never drink your full daily dose gulping it in short period of time. It will do more harm to your body than good. The water intake should be gradual, spread over the entire day.

The ideal temperature of water for drinking is room temperature. When the water is too hot or too cold, it takes much more energy for the body to be able to use that water. It will also be much easier for you to fulfill you daily water dose with slightly warm water because is much more drinkable.

I do not recommend drinking water during exercise. I do recommend however, finishing 1 glass of plain water at least 30 minutes before exercise and 5 – 10 minutes after exercise (after your heartbeat has slowed down to a normal pace).

As much as we stress-out the importance of water, there is one ingredient that should always go along with water – *salt*.

Salt

It is well known that water and light make the life possible; however, there are many people that may be very surprised to hear that salt is another ingredient without which life would not exist, at least on this planet. You may probably hear some people say that salt is "white death" (as well as sugar). It cannot be any further from the truth. Life began not just in water, it began in **salt** water of the ocean.

For thousands of years of human civilization salt was one of the most precious commodities that was traded as precious stones and was admired by many cultures and religions not only for its flavor-adding qualities, but mostly for its health related qualities. Salt was so valuable that it was, quite literally, worth it's weight in gold. If you would explore the history of salt, you would be surprised how interesting it is. Salt truly affected the history of the world.

There are numerous properties of salt we could talk about, but I will mention just some – enough for you to understand its importance. Salt can be used as a remedy for treating conditions that include asthma, Alzheimer disease, stress, depression, high blood pressure, diabetes, and many others. Salt's functions in the body include supporting strength and condition of all muscles, bones strength and their structure, improving sleep, balancing the level of sugar in the blood, it is absolutely necessary for production of hydro-electricity in all cells, transferring information between nerve cells in the brain, absorption of food we eat, and probably the most important function – salt together with potassium (more about potassium later) regulates the amount of water stored in the body.

I want to stress-out the importance of the last mentioned function because it is fully corresponds with previous chapter about water. As much as important the amount of water that we drink, it is actually irrelevant without salt. ***It is the salt and water balance that makes our bodies to function properly***. You can drink lots of water, but if you have no salt in your diet, body cells will not be able to absorb that water, which will simply drain-out with urination and your body will dehydrate.

Those people that say: "salt is harmful" are partially right because salt is harmful **if** it is consumed without enough water. Therefore, we are arriving to a conclusion that water without salt and salt without water are harmful. Only the right balance will help our body to grow taller, stronger and healthier.

How to calculate your daily salt intake:

1.5 – 2 grams of salt (1/4 of a teaspoon) for every 1.2 liters or 5 caps of water.

You should take into account the amount of salt in the food that you eat, as well as liquids other than plain water that you drink. It is usually not easy to find exactly the right balance, but you should not worry if you drink water and eat salt at least approximately according to suggestions in this book. The body will find that balance by itself. The way it works – the salt holds enough water in the body to function properly, at the same time the water washes away extra salt that may be harmful to the body.

Regardless of all benefits, keep in mind that salt that is good for the body is not just any salt. The general rule is – the less processed salt is – the better.

The quality of available salt is very variable. The most balanced and healthy salt comes from evaporated seawater – *natural sea salt*. It may have a slightly gray color, which indicates the presence of a variety of mineral salts other than sodium chloride. Processed salt has just two minerals, while unprocessed natural salt has hundreds. Some of these minerals are calcium, iron, magnesium, potassium, and sodium. They are essential for your body's development.

Most salt sold in grocery stores is processed, and is almost 100 percent made of sodium and chloride. For the purpose of preventing iodine deficiencies, salt manufacturers add iodine to processed salts. Adding iodine to sodium chloride crystals causes them to turn purple. Since purple salt is not common and may look unattractive, the salt is bleached to turn it white again. Flow agents (chemicals) are also added to reduce the absorption of moisture from the air to keep the salt flowing from your saltshaker. As you can see, most table salt is no longer in its natural form. It has had all the minerals except sodium and chloride removed and it contains residues of the bleaching chemicals, along with the flow agents. Major producing companies dry their salt in huge kilns with temperatures reaching 1200 degrees F, changing he salt's chemical structure, which in turn adversely affects the human body. Fish from the ocean will die quickly if placed in a solution of refined salt and water. The sodium chloride, in its form as it comes from the refinery, is actually poisonous to fish, which means it is *poisonous humans too.*

Also understand that refined iodized salt is often hidden in processed foods. Salt is a cheap way to make food tasty and is used liberally in producing packaged and fast food. Avoiding the excess salt in processed foods is just one more important reason for eating plenty of fresh, natural foods and less processed foods.

Sea salt, usually sold in health food stores, also may have had all the minerals except sodium and chloride removed. If a salt is very white and dry, it has had the additional minerals removed. In its natural form, salt is usually grayish, or off-white, and is moist.

When buying salt read packaging carefully and if possible buy "unprocessed" or "certified organic" sea salt. Use those brands that are as unrefined as possible with minimal processing. Most of the labels on salt packages will indicate that, but if the label doesn't mention the production method, it's a safe bet that the salt is heavily processed.

An easy way to check if the salt was processed is to mix a spoonful of salt in a glass of water and let it stand overnight. If the salt collects at the bottom of the glass after many hours in the water – it has been processed. Salt that will not dissolve in water cannot dissolve in your body. Any foreign substance that collects in the body organs and tissues will eventually result in malfunctioning of essential body processes.

I want to stress-out one more time the importance of the *water/salt balance.* If you are not drinking enough water, overuse of salt is dangerous for health. It can be a factor in the development of cardiovascular disease, high blood pressure and even stroke. Excessive use of salt causes the kidneys to work harder in order to process it. Overuse of salt can be very harmful and even fatal to very small children. The best way to avoid the over consumption of salt is to drink water as described above and prepare meals at home. Try to avoid purchasing foods that are only available in cans, avoid or at lease limit fast food restaurants.

Keep in mind that if you use salt without iodine, you have to include iodine, a necessary nutrient, in your diet. A great source or iodine is seaweed. By the way, seaweed is one of the most nutritious and most powerful anti-oxidants foods on Earth. Along with iodine, it is rich in vitamins and minerals such as calcium, magnesium, potassium, iron and zinc as well as vitamins C, B1, B2, B6 and B12. Yogurt, cow's milk, mozzarella cheese, eggs, and strawberries are also good sources of iodine.

There are many types of salt that are available on the market, however all of them at some point of time came from the ocean. The difference between types of salt depends on what location on the planet salt came from and how it was produced and processed. Salt is produced using three methods: rock salt mining, solar evaporation, and vacuum evaporation. Salt is primarily found underground in rock form or dissolved in the world's oceans and some lakes. Salt is also found on the surface of ancient evaporated seabeds. It does matter how the salt was mined or evaporated. Its quality diminishes substantially if it is mined using explosives, or unnaturally evaporated (vacuum evaporation). If you are really serious about treating your body in the best possible manner, use salt that was mined without using explosion methods or produced by natural evaporation under the sun. Your body will thank you for that with great health and greater chance to gain height. It is usually not always easy to find out how the salt was produced, but if you know the source, you can usually dig-out the way of production. Also, if the salt was produced by good methods, it is usually mentioned on the label.

Remember: **water and salt are necessary ingredients your body needs to develop and grow.**

Sleep

Bedtime is the time when we grow the most, and the amount of growth each night depends on how you prepare your body during the day. Have you ever checked your height before going to sleep and then again right after you woke up the next morning? If not, try it. You will see that in the morning you will be taller than in the evening. You might be amazed when you see the difference, which can be as little as 1/4 of an inch, and as much as two inches, sometimes even more. The reason for this miracle is simple: during the day, when we are in vertical positions, our bones and joints are compressing because of the earth's gravitation. So, in effect, we are growing down until we go to bed. While we sleep (I hope you sleep horizontally) the earth's gravitation does not affect us. Our bones and joints will then decompress and the body's length will increase.

To maximize your night growth time you need to perform exercises shown in this book. On top of all important reasons for performing exercises, your bones and cartilages will not be as compressed as they would have been without an exercise routine. If your bones are very compressed, longer time will be required for them to get decompressed and less time will be left for your body to grow while at sleep.

You should sleep on a firm orthopedic mattress with a small pillow or better yet, with no pillow. You should make sure to get enough sleep every night in order to maximize the bones decompression effect and growth hormone release.

Optimally, you should sleep 8 – 10 hours every day. I do not recommend sleeping for more than 10 hours at night; however if you will be able to find at least a few minutes or up to an hour of additional sleep time during the day (siesta – a common tradition in some countries and cultures), it will be very beneficial to your body's growth and to your health in general.

As mentioned in a chapter "Human Growth Hormone", growth hormone is more actively produced during the night than during the day, allowing the body to grow faster. The most active growth hormone release occurs during deep level sleep, which starts about 90 minutes after you go to sleep. In order for you to prolong the hormone release period, you need to prolong the deep level sleep.

How to achieve deep level sleep:

◆ Sleeping on your back with a small pillow under your knees (assuming that you sleep on a firm orthopedic mattress) will prevent any backaches that may cause you not even getting deep sleep, among other negative effects on your health.

◆ Keep your hands and feet warm, wear comfortable clothes.

◆ Sleep in a dark and quiet room.

◆ Go to sleep at the same time every day (I know – it's difficult, especially on weekends, but try your best).

◆ Drink a glass of pure clean water right before going to sleep (see chapter "Water").

As you go to sleep, practice total relaxation. Close your eyes and breathe deeply as follows: inhaling through the nose for 4 seconds, hold your breath for 6 seconds, then slowly exhaling through the mouth for 10 seconds. Do this 5 times. Then concentrate your thought on your brain, think of it as a muscle and start slowly to relax it as a muscle for about a minute or two. As your brain relaxes, you will start feeling very light energy concentration in the brain. That energy concentration or substance is a part of your energy twin (read chapter "The Power Of Thought"). It is liquid and can easily be moved by your thought throughout your body, even outside. Imagine this light liquid energy slowly flowing down from the brain past your forehead, eyes, and mouth to the neck. As the liquid energy moves, you will feel it as a warm and soothing sensation. After going through the neck, move the energy into the right arm, lowly reaching your fingers, then back towards your left arm. After traveling through the left arm and coming back to the chest area, stop the liquid energy there, thinking how it expands filling-up the entire upper portion of you torso. As you feel every organ and tissue of your upper body bathe in this worm light liquid of energy, very slowly move the energy down through your body, through both legs, exiting outside your body through your feet, completely dissolving there.

You may repeat this mental exercise several times until falling asleep. You may also not feel this energy when trying it for the first time, but trust me, this energy exist. As you repeat the exercise many times, your body will become more sensitive to this experience and you will start feeling the sensation of the liquid energy flowing through your body. This will create the best possible condition for you pituitary gland to release the maximum amount of growth hormone into your body during night sleep.

Another great thing you can do – right before you go to sleep, hang relaxed on the chin-up bar for as long as you can. Do not do any exercise; just try to be as relaxed as you can.

An important study was made by researchers at Albert Einstein College of Medicine of Yeshiva University. According to their research, snoring and other nighttime breathing problems could stunt a child's growth. Please read some excerpt from their article published in November 2008:

"As many as one in five children experience breathing problems during sleep, such as snoring, mouth breathing, and apnea (abnormally long pauses in respiration). Researchers have long suspected these problems – collectively known as sleep disordered breathing (SDB) – contribute to growth delays in children. SDB interrupts deep sleep, a period of the sleep cycle when the body typically secretes large amounts

of growth hormone. Children with SDB are thought to produce a lesser amount of growth hormone".

"These studies involved children with enlarged tonsils and/or adenoids – the principal causes of SDB. (Other causes of SDB include obesity, neuromuscular weakness of airway muscles, and craniofacial abnormalities.) All the children had their tonsils/ adenoids surgically removed, either to treat symptoms of SDB or recurrent infection, or both. They were then monitored to measure the impact of the surgery – which is usually curative – on growth".

"Our meta-analysis found significant increases in both standardized height and weight following surgery," says Dr. Bonuck, whose paper was published online by Archives of Disease in Childhood. "In other words, while all the children were expected to continue to grow after they underwent surgery, their growth rates were much greater than expected."

These results are particularly important because studies show that only one in two pediatricians is aware of any potential link between SDB and growth failure. "Our findings suggest that primary-care providers and specialists should consider the possibility of SDB when they see children with growth failure," says Dr. Bonuck.

"For parents, the take-home message is to be alert to symptoms of SDB, particularly habitual snoring, which tend to peak during the preschool years. Such monitoring may help prevent growth delays in children from occurring in the first place, she says."

"Growth delays are not the only reason why parents need to be attuned to SDB symptoms, adds Dr. Bonuck. SDB is also associated with increased risk of behavioral or cognitive issues, such as attention-deficit hyperactivity disorder (ADHD) and other learning disabilities."

As you can see from this report, a simple treatment of a sleep disorder can increase the release of growth hormone and make a child grow taller. This can be done at a fraction of the cost of any man-made growth hormone therapy (which I do not recommend anyway as was described above in the chapter "Human Growth Hormone").

There are certain stressful conditions that are also blocking the release of growth hormone during sleep, such as depression, anxiety and other psychological problems. If you feel depressed, something bothers you for any reason, you wake-up many times at night or just cannot sleep – you really need to improve your state of mind if you are serious about your health and height.

First of all, I would advise you to read again the "State of your awareness and mood" section in the "Human Growth Hormone" chapter of this book. I clearly explained there how easy it is to improve your mood and keep it that way. Let me also add that regardless of what your situation is, regardless of how complicated and difficult it is, I can guarantee you that there are always ways out of any situation. And if you do not see the way out of your difficult situation, it's just because you did not search for it good enough. More often than not, the best way to deal with a difficult situation is to accept things the way they are, as your normal reality, and then deal with it gradually improving things as you move along.

As we discussed previously in the book, you are – who you think you are, so just think of an ideal person that you would want to be, try to be an actor and play the role as if you are that person. If you will do it long enough, I can assure you – you **will** become that person! Your thoughts do materialize, remember? Moreover, *every difficult situation in life is just an opportunity to learn from it, and is always the greatest opportunity to make an important change in your life.*

Did you know that most accomplishments in human history were made only after some negative events happened that pushed people to make those accomplishments?

Deal with your stress and sleep tight, you can do it.

Pay close attention to the quality of your sleep and you will be rewarded well. If you have the sleep disordered breathing, you may not know about it as you cannot check this yourself while sleeping. You can ask your parents to check on you while you are at sleep. You can also record yourself during the night by an audio recorder with voice activation. It will record only snoring and other noises you will produce. If you suspect having sleep disordered breathing, definitely check-up with your doctor, it can make a big difference.

Affects of Sunlight

You probably know that all plants need sunlight to grow and survive. But what about animals and people? We all know that without Sun there would be no life on this planet, still many of us unfortunately forgot or never even thought that all of us truly need that sunlight to live.

> *Sunlight is the source and the engine of every living creature on this planet (except some organisms at the bottom of deep ocean that live on heat from lava and the bacteria). Everything that happens to us, including the way we are and the way we live, fully depends on Sun and its activities.*

As much as we depend on it, majority of people especially in big cities rarely stay under sunlight. Just over 100 years ago, before the light bulb got into our households, people spent over 90% of their daytime outside under the sun. That was the case for as long as people walked on this planet. For millions of years our bodies depended on being under the sun most of the time, and it was considered as torture to place a person in a room with no sunlight for long time. Now, 10% or less of sunlight is the norm for many of us. That is one of the big reasons for health problems in our civilization. We need sun now just like we needed it 100 or so years ago. Its *ultraviolet light plays a huge role in our body's processes*. If you want to be healthy, if you want your body to develop properly and grow taller, you need to remember that.

I don't believe that just telling you what to do will make you do it; I believe that *you should know reasons behind my words*. I want you to understand and believe in what you do. That is why the following information will be very helpful.

Did you know that light has physical properties, and it is part of all living organisms? Yes, every little cell in our body is filled with light, even if we are in full darkness. This light is very dim. If we would look at each cell with microscope, the light would seem like looking at a candle light from 20 miles away. Still, this light exists and plays a major role in every process of the body. This light travels throughout the body through special "highways" called "meridians", energetically connecting different organs with each other and providing the exchange of information between cells with the speed of light. All meridians in the body are connected with the surface of the body in hundreds of points called "acupuncture points". These points are used in Chinese medicine for thousands of years to diagnose and treat many diseases. What is interesting – when we are under the sun, the sunlight enters the body through these acupuncture points, traveling deep inside through meridians just like through optical fibers, and feeding the "interior light supply" of every cell in every organ.

Now, as you understand that the light not only touches our skin, but also goes through the skin reaching every organ, you should understand why the light affects every process in the body. If the body is not developing as it should, if a person gets sick often, one of the main reasons is that there is not enough light stored in the body. As the consequence, the exchange of information between cells is disturbed, which in turn disturbs all biological processes leading to many malfunctions, *including stunned body's growth.*

Let me stress-out an important fact: many studies have shown that **children grow faster in the spring and summer than in the autumn and winter.** Not only studies, almost all parents who check their children's height periodically, will tell you that they have noticed such difference, and often it is very significant. Why do you think is that? Don't you like to get outside more often when the weather is nice? Of course, during the spring and summer kids are exposed the most to the sunlight. It is the increased exposure to the sun that makes our bodies grow faster during those periods. As explained above, when our body is filled with light – all its processes are functioning properly, and body's development is at its best.

The fact is – people who live in darkness suffer from infectious diseases, have soft and porous bones, depression, chronic body pain, diabetes, respiratory and other disorders, as well as decreasing the body's development process.

You are probably questioning why is only sunlight so beneficial, what about the light produced by electricity? The answer is simple: it is the ultraviolet light produced by sun what makes it so useful. Regular electricity light sources do not produce spectrum that would be enough for us, only Sun radiates what our bodies need. We will not get into too much detail, it is not a science book after all, but the basics will not hurt to know. Sunlight is not just light, the Sun radiates many very different types of waves, a very wide spectrum of them. This spectrum consists of visible light, ultraviolet light, and infrared light. Each of them has wide spectrum as well. Ultraviolet light is invisible and takes only about 10% of the entire spectrum, but it affects our bodies the most.

Ultraviolet light affects can be positive and negative, depending on longevity and type of exposure to the Sunlight. Ultraviolet light kills bad viruses and bacteria, prevents infections, prevents the development of some cancers, strengthen the immune system, necessary for health of our eyes, helpful in correcting blood pressure, kidney problems and skin diseases, necessary for the organism to heal itself, and it also *triggers the production of vitamin D, which plays very important role in the calcium digestion.*

We will discuss more about calcium later in the book, I will just mention that calcium is the main mineral that supports the structure of our bones, and it makes them strong. Also, calcium promotes the growth and strength of our muscles. The interesting fact is that without vitamin D calcium cannot properly function. Basically, *calcium and vitamin D are the "partners" in growing your bones and muscles*, and keeping them that way. As information for an older person reading this, know that lack of Vitamin D may increase the risk of lung cancer, Parkinson disease, diabetes, and high blood pressure.

Keep in mind that vitamin D is not only produced by the exposure to the sun, it also contains in different foods (much more on that later in the book), and it is also available in supplements. Food and supplement sources are good but not enough for the body, you should always combine them with sunbath.

> *Putting it all together, we will come to the conclusion that on top of all the benefits sunlight provides for the body's protection and development, it helps grow and strengthen your bones and muscles, giving the power and strength to your body.*

It is also very important to know that the overexposure to ultraviolet light and overheating could cause skin burn and even skin cancer. We will discuss later how to prevent that.

Now as you understand the importance of being under the Sun as well as its dangers, lets discuss what to do to reap the most benefits from the Sun without any negative consequences. *I cannot stress enough the importance of the following, so please read on.*

Rules to Sun exposure

First and most important rule – never stay under hot sun for longer then several minutes if you are not prepared. I guarantee – you will regret it.

During cold periods of the year the rule is simple – stay outside as often as you can, just avoid constant sunlight exposure for over 2 – 3 hours when the sky is clear and Sun is at its peak.

The hotter the sun gets, the more careful you should be exposing to the direct sunlight. During the summer, the best possible sunlight you should be exposed to is in the morning, usually before 11 AM when it is completely harmless and most beneficial. Try to get outside as early as possible, especially for your morning exercise routine (later on that). Evenings are also best to be spent outside. During the day, when the sunlight is at its hottest, it is still best to spend time outside, only in the shadow. Even in a shadow the Sun's energy reaches you, activating your body's metabolism.

If you did not expose yourself to a hot Sun for at least a month, and all-of-a-sudden start spending a lot of time under the sun, you may do great harm to your body. Start only with a few minutes of direct sunlight exposure in the first day. Increase the timing very gradually adding only a few minutes to the total direct daytime Sun exposure each day. If you do it this way, your skin and your entire body will successfully adopt to a much longer direct sunlight exposure. You will not even need to use any sunblock or sunscreen products to protect yourself from getting sunburn, except maybe the most sensitive areas such as the nose and the ears.

Speaking of sunblock and sunscreen products, you should know that using them does not mean you are fully protected from getting high levels of ultraviolet (UV) radiation. It is also well known that these products do not prevent from getting skin cancer, which may not necessarily appear right away, but many years after overexposure. It means that *if you stay under burning Sun for a long time even fully covered with powerful sunscreen, especially when unprepared – you may still badly suffer from this later on in your life.* Moreover, many sunblock and sunscreen products may contain chemicals that are not necessarily healthy for your skin and body, and may also do damage if used excessively.

Regardless of negatives, you should still use sunscreen if you chose to be under the burning Sun for long time with little clothes on, especially if your skin is unprepared. I do recommend however to always cover your body with clothes (cotton is usually the best) when you are exposed to the hot sun at its peak. Always cover your head. When you feel burning sensation on the skin, it is a good indicator that you should cover yourself or go into the shadow.

Did you know that all the blood in the body travels very close to our eyes? It means that gelling lots of light into your eyes feeds your entire blood supply and your entire body with very much needed light. This does not mean you should stare at the sun, you may damage your eyes this way; *just look at bright objects that are exposed to the sunlight*. The only time when you can stare directly at the sun is at the sunrise and sunset. It is actually an *extremely powerful way to get a good boost to your body's internal processes*. The way to do it: look at the sun with one eye closed for a few seconds, then switch eyes. Repeat several times, each following time increasing the exposure by 3 – 5 seconds. Do not over-do it, if you feel uncomfortable – stop right away.

Everything that we eat and drink has energy; part of this energy is the energy of light. Consuming foods that are full of light is another way to acquire the necessary reserve of light. The problem with this is that most of the foods that we buy at stores have no or very little energy of light left in them, because it disappears when the food is processed or even when it is frozen. Only fruits, vegetables, berries and mushrooms that were recently picked and never stored in a dark freezer have plenty of light energy and are the best for consumption. If you don't have the luxury of having truly fresh unprocessed foods, you need even more sunlight in your life. The same rule applies to the water. *The water that was exposed to the direct sunlight is well energized and is great for our bodies*. To energize the pure water with the sunlight, store it in a clear glass jar and place it outside under direct sunlight for at least a day. If you do that, *this water will be your secret weapon in your quest to gain height*.

You should also understand that enough sunlight alone is not enough for proper development and growth, everything else mentioned in this book is very important to follow as well. *Don't forget that the fresh air that you breathe outside also plays an important role. We need oxygen from the fresh air for the body to function, develop, and grow properly.* This will lead us to the subject – breathing.

Breathing

Breathing is synonymous with life. Yet, for most of us it is just one more of those things that we take for granted. After all, it is just about inhaling oxygen and exhaling carbon dioxide, right? Wrong. Let me show you what I mean and what it has to do with body's development and growth.

Everything that we do, how we feel, and the way our bodies develop fully depend on how we breathe. You don't believe me, try to change your breathing pattern (breath slower or faster) at least for a minute, and then think again. If you feel a big difference even within one minute, can you imagine how much the body can be affected if a person's breathing pattern will permanently change even a little? That is why incorrect breathing always negatively affects every process in our body as well as its development and growth. In fact, poor breathing causes or worsens chronic maladies such as asthma, allergies, anxiety, fatigue, depression, headaches, heart conditions, high blood pressure, sleep loss, obesity, harmful stress, poor mental clarity plus hundreds of other lesser known but equally harmful conditions. Moreover, *all diseases are caused or worsened by poor breathing*.

Now, as you understand the importance of it, let's see if you are breathing correctly. Place one hand on your tummy, the other on your chest. Take a deep breath in and see which hand moves out. If your abdomen expands when you inhale and air seems to flow in deeply to the bottom of your stomach, you're on the right track. However, if your lower abdomen expands when you exhale and compresses when you inhale, you are a shallow breather, which is not good. Pulling in your stomach as you inhale creates tension and wastes energy. Squeezing the abdomen pushes the diaphragm upward, minimizing your lungs' capacity, simultaneously pushing and fighting against the inflow of every breath.

> *While you are young and in good health, these bits of wasted effort and restrained oxygen intake may not seem apparent, but over time, exhaustion and tension will take their toll on your mental, physical and emotional well-being.*

Therefore, *the right way to breathe-in is through the nose, slowly filling the stomach with air first, and then slowly filling the chest. Breath-out slowly through the nose or mouth, squeezing the air out of the stomach first, then from the chest.* This abdominal breathing pulls the air down into the deepest parts of the lungs where the air exchange is most efficient.

Without underestimating the importance of abdominal breathing, I should also stress-out the importance of having the right balance of oxygen and carbon dioxide – two ingredients without which we cannot survive even for few minutes. The air we breathe is a mixture of gases that include oxygen, carbon dioxide, nitrogen, water, argon and trace gases. Oxygen's portion of that mixture is about 21%. When oxygen gets into our lungs, the blood picks it up with its red blood cells, spreading it throughout into every cell in the body. At the same time, these red blood cells are giving-up the excess carbon dioxide gas that was picked-up from all the cells in the body. Basically, all the cells in the body use the oxygen delivered by the blood to produce energy they need to survive and reproduce, and the carbon dioxide is a byproduct of that chemical reaction, which plays an important role in the process of releasing oxygen into blood cells. As you can see, *carbon dioxide and oxygen work together as equal partners that need each other.*

To grow and function properly, the body needs only certain amount of oxygen to process. If it gets too much or too little oxygen on the regular basis, the body will eventually adapt to it and you will think you breathe normally, but in reality all your organs will suffer and will not function as well as they could, which in the short run will *reduce your body's growth*, and in the long run will substantially diminish your health and reduce your lifespan.

So, how do we control the right balance of oxygen and carbon dioxide? *By the amount of air we breathe-in and how long we hold it inside.* Te rule is – the deeper and faster we breathe, the more oxygen and less carbon dioxide we get, the slower we breathe, the more carbon dioxide and less oxygen we get.

First, lets do two simple tests to see if you breathe correctly, and if the balance of oxygen and carbon dioxide is normal or not:

◆ Sit-down comfortably in a chair till you are fully relaxed and breathing normally, then count how many respirations you do in one minute, using the stopwatch. The younger you are – the more breaths per minute you should have. On average, it can be as high as 44 breaths per minute in infants and as low as 10 breaths per minute in adults. Teenagers should expect 14 – 25 breaths per minute. It is considered as good rate to have 12 respirations per minute for adults of over 25 years old, however if you are an adult reading this, I strongly recommend trying to gradually reduce this rate down to 8 or even 6 per minute as it will greatly improve your energy level and general health increasing you lifespan. See below for techniques.

◆ Sit-down comfortably in a chair till you are fully relaxed and breathing normally, then inhale and hold the breath for as long as you can while using the stopwatch to count how many seconds you can hold the breath. Less than 15 seconds shows extremely low level of carbon dioxide in the blood and is not good, 15 – 30 seconds still bad, 30 – 45 seconds is a norm, 45 – 60 seconds show very good balance, over 60 seconds is excellent.

If the second test showed that the level of carbon dioxide in your blood is very good, most likely your respiratory rate is the way it should be and you should do nothing to improve it. If the level of carbon dioxide is lower than should be, then your respiratory rate most likely is too rapid, and should be decreased.

There are many techniques to reduce the number of respirations, but we will discuss only several simple and very effective techniques:

◆ One technique is called "4-7-8 Breathing" in which you inhale to the count of four, hold the breath to the count of seven, and slowly exhale to the count of eight. Keep in mind that *slow exhale* is key. Remember to keep yourself fully relaxed.

◆ Technique "3-9-6": inhale to the count of three, slowly exhale to the count of nine, and hold the breath to the count of six. If it is too difficult, reduce counts to "3-6-4". If it is easy for you, try to increase exhale and holding time by 1 second or more. Do this technique and the one above for 3 – 5 minutes, repeating 3 times per day on the first week and 5 times per day on the second week and thereafter. Continue for up to a month, increasing exhale and holding time by 1 – 2 seconds each week. You can mix both techniques as you please.

◆ Breathe normally and relaxed for a minute, then exhale and hold the breath for as long as you can, slowly inhale, then hold the breath to for several seconds till you feel comfortable. Repeat 3 – 5 times with 1 minute rest in between, 3 – 5 times each day. Each day try to increase holding time by 1 – 2 seconds. This may not be easy, but it is very effective, moreover there is one extremely powerful benefit to that technique: ***it will seriously boost the release of growth hormone*** by the pituitary gland!

All above breathing techniques should not be performed during or after meal times and exercises as they may do more damage than good.

I understand, you may think that this is not an easy task if you were breathing incorrectly for most of your life. It will not be hard at all if you will make it your goal and stay focused.

All newborn babies breathe correctly; it's just many of us gradually and unintentionally change the way we breathe because of our changed lifestyles such as limited mobility, lack of physical activity, over-eating, hot days and overheated stuffy rooms.

> *You should open all the windows and doors every-day to air the house off.*

Physical posture and tense muscles can also greatly affect breathing. In other words, even if you have perfect posture but stiff statue, proper breathing is not possible. We need to keep our body flexible and relaxed. You will accomplish that by following exercises and massage techniques you will learn in following chapters.

The "trick" is to remember to practice your breathing and to perform it correctly. With time, these skills become your normal method of breathing, you just need to be a little bit patient.

As we learned in the last breathing technique (exhale and holding the breath), one powerful thing you can do with breathing – increasing the release of growth hormone. This works on the same principal as resistance or high-intensity exercises described earlier in the chapter "Human Growth Hormone". The difference is that you can do breathing technique more often than high-intensity exercises. Too much of anything is no good, and this rule applies to this breathing technique as well, so do it without creating too much stress to your body. Usually 20 – 30 times within a day is more than enough.

Even though I prefer exhaling technique for growth hormone release, you can also do inhaling instead. Just inhale and hold the breath for as long as you can, then very slowly release the air. Very important – do not breath heavily after that; try to gradually calm your thirst for oxygen down.

There is one extremely powerful activity you can do that may do wonders to your heights increase. This simple activity combines breathing technique, high-intensity exercises, stimulating almost all growth plates and spinal discs, and stretching muscles – the maximum package you can imagine. This activity is – swimming under water. We will discuss more about swimming later in this book where you will learn how swimming is great for our bodies' growth, as well as how to swim under water. Just remember that swimming, especially underwater can be dangerous, so always be very careful and never do anything risky – it's not worth it.

Massage

I'm sure you know the feeling of when you really need someone to touch you. There were many researches made on this subject that proved how important touch can be for anyone. Touch is a necessity for a healthy life, and good massage is the healthiest touch of all.

We may not think of it as a regular necessity, but massage has a long and historical list of benefits for every person at every age. Not only it is relaxing, but also healing and nurturing, stimulating growth and rejuvenating. Massage can be a very welcome alternative treatment for many causes of pain. Here are some facts about massage:

- Infants born prematurely who receive infant massage gain more weight and leave the hospital 50% sooner.

- For older individuals, massage helps keeping joints mobile, helps stimulate the skin and improve circulation, improves range of motion and reduces pain.

- Massage reduces recovery time from injuries and surgery, reduces swelling and scar tissue, releases endorphins, reduces anxiety, fatigue and stress, boosts the immune system, stimulates lymph flow and detoxification, reduces stiffness, improves sleep, reduces neck pain, back pain, sciatica, tendonitis, headaches, shoulder pain, and much, much more.

- Massage makes a healthy person even healthier. Helpful touch not only feels good, but also is good for us.

- The most important benefit for us in the scope of this book is that ***massage therapy stimulates growth hormone release***. This is especially important for very young children.

For parents of a newborn baby I strongly suggest to give their baby massage every day. It will most definitely stimulate baby's development and growth. There are many books written about baby massage and I suggest parents to read one or two, and familiarize themselves with techniques before performing massage on their little ones. It is important to understand that wrongly performed massage can easily do harm to babies. Lets look at just few simple safe techniques.

Some of baby massage techniques:

- Put a few drops of baby oil on your palms and rub hands together to warm them-up and spread the oil.

- Rubbing the back: place your hands down on the baby's back and massage (move the muscles beneath the skin) in gentle, circular motions.

- Milking the limbs: grab the top of the thigh of top of arm and place your hands around it. Make slow, firm strokes down toward the ankles or wrists.

- Rolling motions: place your hands perpendicular on one of your baby's limbs. Roll your hands back and forth as if making a snake out of dough.

For you, my young feller is not necessary to ask your parents or someone else to give you a massage because you can do it yourself. Don't get me wrong, the massage done well by another person is better than self-massage. It's just with self-massage you don't have to rely on someone every time; you can do it at any time of your convenience.

We have two purposes for the massage:

1. To stimulate all your organs so that they will perform at their best. Without getting into much detail, you should simply understand that a healthy organism develops and grow better. All organs and all little cells in our body are connected and fully dependent on each other. One poorly performing organ will affect, in some extent, all other organs in your body. That is why you need massage to stimulate your entire body. It is not hard, just read further.

2. To stimulate the pituitary gland in order to *increase the release of growth hormone* among other important hormones. This was already fully described in the chapter "Human Growth Hormone" earlier in this book.

Massage is a very complex field, and professionals spend years to study and master it. But we don't want to spend years to learn it, we want to learn it and use it today, *we want some shortcuts*. That is why I will give you very basic but very powerful shortcuts to stimulate every organ in your body. These shortcuts are: your **feet**, **hands** and **ears**.

The surface of our feet, hands and ears has hundreds of very small areas, each connected with a particular organ in the body by a tiny energy channel. These areas are called *reflect points*. When the reflect point is stimulated or massaged, it automatically stimulates the organ it is connected with.

There are hundreds of reflect points, and for best results each should be stimulated separately, however we definitely will not do that in the scope of this program (except working on couple of reflex areas that was described the chapter "Human Growth Hormone", section "Stimulating reflex areas"). Instead, all we have to do is to use simple massage techniques and still getting great results.

Feet massage

It's easy to massage your feet by sitting on a chair and resting one foot on the opposite leg. If you like, you can rub some massage oil or lotion onto your foot. It is best to massage your feet without socks.

1. Start by lightly rubbing your leg, sliding your hands from foot up to the ankle and back down to the foot – several times.

2. Place your thumb on top of the other and firmly press down the center of your sole on either side. With one thumb, do continuously circular pressures on the arch and ball of the foot.

3. Apply pressure with your thumbs to the sole of your foot, working from the bottom of your arch to the top near your big toe. Repeat five times.

4. Support your foot with one hand and make a loose fist with the other. Do knuckle movements all throughout your sole and also ripple your fingers around in small, circular movements.

5. Massage each toe by holding it firmly and moving it from side to side. Extend each toe gently out and away from the ball of your foot. Then apply pressure to the areas between your toes.

6. Hold your toes in one hand and bend them backward holding them there for five to ten seconds. Then bend them in the opposite direction and hold for five to ten seconds. Repeat three times.

7. Use your thumbs to press and move in small circles along the sole of the foot. Cover the entire surface of the sole.

8. Squeeze your foot hard along its length.

9. Switch feet and repeat. Enjoy your foot rub repeating each step above several times.

Hand massage

1. Stroke the back of your hand, pushing firmly up toward the wrist and gliding back gently. Squeeze the hand all over, pressing between the palm and fingers.

2. Squeeze each finger, starting near the palm and gradually working back to the tip, pulling and gently stretching it; gently rock your finger as you do this. Continue to grip up the finger and off the tip.

3. Squeeze the little flap of skin between the fingers.

4. Link your hands together; fingers grasping fingers but keeping them straight, then squeeze your fingers together, rotate them while doing this.

5. Still with fingers clasped, push your arms straight out in front of you, so your fingers are strongly extended and your shoulders are pulled forward.

6. Stroke between the tendons on the back of your hand with your thumb. Complete four strokes in each furrow continuing to the wrists.

7. Turn your hand over and support the back with your fingers. Complete circular pressure with the thumb, pressing deeply and continuing throughout your palm and end at the wrist.

8. Strongly hold one finger at its tip and shake it hard so your entire hand will shake. Do 10 – 15 strokes it for each finger, or until you will feel as the finger becomes more relaxed as a lifeless rope.

9. Finish by gently stroking the palm of your hand from the tips of your fingers to your wrist.

Ear massage

1. Make circles with your thumbs inside the widest upper part inside the ears, holding them from outside with the two other fingers.

2. Use your forefinger to run inside the ears following their shape upside-down from the part closest to the head. You have to work a little bit with your fingers to place them inside. It is not the main hole but the external one.

3. With your thumbs massage the upper external parts starting from the middle-ear. Keep only the second finger on the other side (like pulling the ear). Press strongly, do it with energy until you start feeling the blood flushing-in and ear becomes hot.

4. Massaging the lobes by gently pulling them down and also making circles with your forefingers and the thumbs, gently and vigorously at the same time. It's really enjoyable, and each hand helps the respective ear. You can also do it by crossing your hands towards the opposite ears.

Immediately after, the ears will be red and you will be able to feel the blood circulation inside of ears and in the brain. Aftermath you'll enjoy a beautiful sense of relaxing and a gently cool breeze tickling around the ears.

All these simple techniques will stimulate the harmony of your entire body, making the progress of your body's growth a pleasurable adventure.

Physical Exercise

Proper exercise is an extremely important part of the program and I'm suggesting to review it carefully and follow as much as you can. The purpose of exercise, beside of all the health benefits, is to literally help your energy twin to accomplish the assignment you gave it, which is to increase the size of your body. I hope you still remember to keep thinking of energy twin, imagining it grow (read chapter "The Power Of Thought").

Exercises I will show you will serve these main purposes: **stimulating growth plates, stimulating spinal discs, relaxing and stretching muscles** that otherwise could stunt body's growth, **strengthening some muscles** that will support body's growth, and **increasing the release of growth hormone.**

Growth plates are parts of the long bones of children and young adults. These plates are areas of growing tissue near the bones' ends. Each long bone has at least two growth plates – one at each end. This is where the long bones grow. When young people finish growing, the growth plates are fused and replaced by solid bone. *Our goal is to stimulate growth plates,* which increases the speed at which the tissue is growing and prolonging its lifespan, before growth plates are completely fused.

Stimulating spinal discs is also very important. Spinal disks are soft cushions that sit between spinal bones (vertebrae), acting as spacers and shock absorbers and responsible for the spine flexibility. Stimulating spinal disks with movements that will be shown later will stimulate growth of spinal bones. It will also increase supply of nutrients, oxygen and water into spinal discs, which will increase their thickness, adding to the total height of your body.

Relaxing and stretching muscles is necessary to provide more freedom for bones to grow. Think of it like this: if your bones are under constant pressure, they will not grow as much as if the pressure were removed. If your muscles are stiff, they create that pressure, even when you lay down. When you relax and stretch your muscles, the pressure disappears and bones are free to grow. Please keep in mind – stretching does not lengthen your bones, it just freeing your bones from the pressure among many other benefits for your health that are also playing very important role in your body's development. You can still build very strong muscles, and at the same time not letting your muscles to stunt your growth. Exercises explained below will help you do just that.

Strengthening some muscles will reduce the pressure on spinal discs and facet joints, helping support all the gains you have accomplished in lengthening your spine.

Some ways to ***increase the release of growth hormone*** with *resistance or high-intensity exercise* were described in the chapter above. As you read further, you will find several particular exercises that are designed to boost the release of growth hormone.

As you became more knowledgeable on what your body needs and why, you are ready to start learning how to perform your physical workout. There are few points that needed to be made before we start. First of all, exercises or active physical activities are absolutely necessary part of this program. Even if you decide to skip something, *don't skip exercise. My main goal is to give you guidance on what muscles and parts of your body you should concentrate on, how you should perform these exercises, and what exercises you should not do.*

I do not believe in strict rules on when these exercises should be performed (with certain limitations explained later) because it is better to do most of these exercises whenever you have time for them than not to do them at all. However, I will structure the exercise routine during the day and during the week in the best possible order for best possible results.

There are no strict rules on how often, what time of the day and for how long you should do all this, however my recommendations for *timing your physical activities and exercise program are as follows:*

- ◆ In order to achieve best results, ideally you will need to exercise every day, but not less than 4 days each week. Even if you skip exercise routine for a day of two, you should still perform recommended later in the book physical activities during the day.

- ◆ Exercise for about 30 – 45 minutes in the morning – 15 minutes after having a glass of water, but 20 minutes before breakfast.

- ◆ Exercise for about 20 – 30 minutes in the evening at least 2 hours before going to sleep.

If you will not do exercises in the morning, you should try to do at lease some of them during the day, and spend more time for exercising in the evening. I strongly recommend, however, that you should find time in the morning because this will give enough energy to your body for the entire day.

> *Your growth plates and spinal discs will be stimulated to grow during the day; certain muscles will be strengthened and stretched in order to support and hold your entire body's accomplishments; your blood will be full of oxygen and will circulate much better, increasing growth hormone level in your blood. That is what you need in order for you to grow.*

It is crucial not to stop the exercise program suddenly, as this should be a continuous process to get results that you want. In other words: the only way for your true success is *not to stop working* on your body until you are satisfied with results.

On the side note, these exercises can be performed at any age, even very old age, and I strongly recommend never to stop if you want to live much longer and happier life.

The entire exercise routine in this book is not only great for achieving all of your growth potential, but is also very good for losing weight, keeping your body in good shape, making your heart work more efficiently, increasing your brain power, making you a strong and a healthy person, and adding many years to your life.

Preparation and tips for exercises

Before starting any exercise, know that from performing exactly the same exercise you can:

◆ get positive results

◆ get no results

◆ bring harm to your body

Results from exercise depend on how clear your goal is, your understanding of why you are doing this, and your mood while performing the exercise. It is very important to understand because *even if you will persistently perform all necessary exercises, but not visualizing results you are doing these exercises for, those results may not even come.* If exercises are performed without belief in any positive results from them and in depressed state, it may actually be damaging to your health. Therefore, *think positive when you exercise* (and at other times), don't forget the lessons from the chapter "The Power Of Thought", visualize your body growing while performing every movement in the exercise routine, think how beneficiary each movement is for your body, think of your ultimate goal and how this exercise is surely moving you towards reaching it.

Keep saying to yourself: I am on my way to accomplish my goal; I am capable of accomplishing anything I can imagine; these exercises do help me grow taller; my body is growing right now. If you are not motivated enough, you will never finish what you need to finish and will never reach your ultimate goal, so always keep yourself motivated. There should be no "ifs" or "maybes", only "I am" and "I do". When you say to yourself "I can", it does not mean you will. To give yourself a much better motivation, keep saying: ***"I am doing it right now"*** – *this is the only thought that does materialize.* Laziness is your worst enemy, do everything you can to keep it away.

When you do exercises, do not make yourself too tired. Just slightly tired is acceptable. Try to keep yourself relaxed at all times. Try not to automate the workout process, always remember your ultimate goal and why these exercises are important.

Do not start the workout if you are too hungry or very tired.

Exercising in rough weather conditions

Exercising in hot and humid or cold and wet weather conditions is challenging and potentially hazardous. When you are prepared, outdoor exercise can be enjoyable and safe during any season.

Tips for exercising in heat and humidity:

◆ Drink more of plain water. Dehydration caused by excessive sweating can lead to heat exhaustion and heat stroke. Drink water before and after exercise even if you don't feel thirsty. As was mentioned previously, I do not recommend water intake during exercise or intense physical activity. Nevertheless, if you

do exercise for extended period of time or feel really thirsty, it is
OK to drink in little doses.

◆   Dress for the heat. Wear loose-fitting, light-colored, and
     lightweight clothes. Cotton is best when sweat-soaked because
     it has a cooling effect.

◆   Use common sense. As a rule, the higher the air temperature,
     the lower the humidity must be to avoid risk of heat injury. For
     example: when air temperature exceeds 80 degrees Fahrenheit
     (26 degrees Celsius), you are at risk if the humidity exceeds
     50%. During very hot and humid spells, you will be better-off
     exercising in cool indoors or go swimming.

◆   Take time to adjust. The body takes time to acclimatize to hot
     weather. It takes 7 to 14 days to fully acclimatize, therefore
     gradually increase your exercise time.

Tips for exercising when it's cold and wet:

◆   Dress in multiple layers of clothing. The outer layer should
     protect you from wind, rain, or snow. Cold temperatures,
     dampness, and wind increase the risk of hypothermia. Sweat
     cools the body quickly during cold weather, while wind
     evaporates it faster. Wear fabrics that insulate and keep
     moisture away. Fabrics made of wool and polypropylene are
     good, while cotton retains moisture.

◆   Protect special body parts like your head, face, hands, and feet.
     Mittens are better than gloves. Cover the head with a wool cap.
     Shield the face with a scarf or high collar. Wear socks that retain
     heat and keep moisture away.

◆   Drink plenty of water. Never drink alcohol before or during a
     workout – it makes the body lose heat faster (I strongly suggest

never to take alcohol at all if you want any good results).

◆ Warm-up indoors before exercising outside. Warming your muscles will also help to prevent injury.

◆ I do not recommend exercising outside if weather conditions are too severe.

Warming-up and Cooling-down

Any exercise routine should never start with the sudden heavy physical stress, and should never suddenly end. Everything should be gradual. Always start with light and easy movements (warming-up), preparing your body for the workload, and always gradually slow down with light and easy movements (cooling-down) at the end.

Warmed-up muscles stretch better and allow greater range of motions for the joints. Also, oxygen easily releases from the blood when muscles are warmed gradually. This prevents you from getting out of breath early. Warming up also improves coordination, burns fat more easily, and reduces abnormal heart responses from sudden exercise.

Cooling-down is just as important as warming-up. This is a process of gradual returning of heart rate and breathing back to normal. If you are serious about your body's development and health, never miss this part of exercise routine.

Warming-up

You need about 5 to 15 minutes to warm-up, depending on how much time you have and intensity of the main exercise routine.

Start with relaxed running at a moderate tempo for several minutes (keep in mind – faster is not better!). Continue with light jumps; do sit-downs (no more than what will make you tired); several times reach the floor with your hands without bending your legs; stretch your body and your arms up as far as you possibly can; curl your upper body left and right while keeping your legs stable; move both arms horizontally to the back then crossing them in the front, pushing as far as possible; quickly rotate both arms vertically.

Remember – your goal should be only to warm-up all muscles in your body. Do not do anything stressful, keep yourself relaxed and try to visualize the entire exercise routine you are about to perform.

Cooling-down

At first, hold your hands together above your head and try to reach as high as possible by stretching all your body, imagine as if someone is trying to pull you up holding your hands. Do it for one minute while you are walking slowly. After that, move your hands in a very slow circular motion up and down without touching each other. Every time your hands rise up, stretch your legs and spine as much as possible. Don't forget – do not stop walking. After 1 – 2 minutes, just continue your slow walk for a few more minutes, relaxing but keeping your posture straight. *Do not forget to keep imagining your energy twin and your body growing as you do that.*

Note: our exercise routine will have many movements that can be used for resistance or high-intensity exercise. As we discussed previously, high-intensity exercises are important parts of our program because they help releasing large amounts of growth hormone into the body. Every such movement in this program has a note that it can be used for such purpose. As mentioned previously, you should do *only* limited amount of high-intensity exercises per day (see section "Resistance or high-intensity exercise" in the chapter "Human Growth Hormone"). That is why you should just select any few that you prefer.

In addition, high-intensity exercise can be performed outside of your regular exercise routine. Good examples of this are power walking or sprint.

Main Exercise routine

Exercise routine can be performed outdoors or indoors, any time of the day, but preferably in the morning.

This routine is divided into four parts: **spinal column workout**, **legs and arms workout**, **chin-up bar workout**, and **jumps**.

Spinal column workout

This is the most important physical workout in this program, so please read it carefully, and try to *follow in order it is shown*. This workout is designed to stimulate every single point of your spinal column, and is very powerful. This workout can be performed anywhere and any time as long as you follow my suggestions above.

Our goal is to stimulate every part of the entire spinal column by bending, compressing, decompressing, and twisting. Entire workout may take you about 25 minutes. We will start working from top of the spine and will end at the bottom.

While performing these movements, try to keep your thoughts concentrated on the spine, try to feel it, enjoy this feeling.

Neck

Following movements of the neck spinal cord will not only trigger its growth, but will significantly increase your memory and thinking abilities, as well as increased ability of the pituitary gland to release growth hormone.

1. Lightly massage all your neck and shoulders muscles with right and left hands for at least one minute.

2. While holding your body and shoulders straight up, bend you head so one ear will face up. Try to extend your neck as far up from your body as you can for 5 – 10 seconds. It's like trying to touch the ceiling with the ear. Do the same for the other side. Repeat 3 – 5 times.

3. Starting position is holding the neck straight up, then try to touch your chest with your chin, sliding it down as much as you can. Move the head up to the start position. Repeat the move 7 – 9 times.

4. Slowly bend your neck to the back (starting position). Now move the head down trying to hide the neck inside the body, just like a turtle hiding the head inside a shell. From that position slowly move the head to the front, trying to push the chin as low as possible. Move the head to the starting position, relax for few seconds, and repeat the move 7 – 9 times.

5. Keep your entire spine straight, shoulders should not be moved. Slowly pull down your head to the right, trying to touch the shoulder with the ear, then the same to the left. Repeat 7 – 9 times to each side.

6. Slowly bend your head forward then to the back while also turning it lightly to the right and left. Repeat 5 times.

7. Turn your head to the right as far as you can, trying to look behind you (do not over-do-it) and hold it for 5 seconds, then slowly turn to the right and do the same. Repeat 5 times to each side.

8. Massage neck and shoulders muscles for one minute to relax them, and then rotate the head full circle – 5 times in one direction, 5 times to the other. Repeat 3 – 5 times.

All movements should be smooth and careful. Always avoid too much pressure on your neck, try to keep it as relaxed as possible at all times. Following above exercises and keeping you head straight up at all times will help you to accomplish just that.

Upper spinal cord

1. Lock your arms in a crisscross position across the chest; Lower down your chin trying to reach the abdomen. This will bend upper spinal cord forward. Now with arms still locked, slowly bend the spine and the head back as far as you can. Repeat 5 – 7 times.

2. Hold your hands on the neck, apart from each other. Slowly bend your upper body to one side by trying to touch your hips with an elbow, then to another side. Repeat 7 – 9 times.

3. Stand-up straight, holding your entire spine vertical. Now try to reach the floor with your arms without bending. Push arms down as hard as you can for 5 – 10 seconds, compressing your entire spinal cord, then do the opposite by pulling your shoulders and entire spine as far up as possible while keeping your arms straight down. This will decompress the spinal cord. Repeat 5 – 7 times.

4. Hold your arms down, then rotate both of your shoulders simultaneously like rolling two wheels of the car ahead, than towards the back. 10 rotation each direction. Repeat 3 – 5 times.

5. Stand straight with legs in a wide but comfortable position, keeping arms down. Bend your body to the right, sliding the right arm along the leg as far down as you can, hold it for a few seconds then do the same to the left. Repeat 7 – 9 times.

6. Stand straight with legs in a wide but comfortable position. Put your hands on shoulders or hold the neck, spreading bended

arms apart. Now turn your upper body together with arms and the head to the right then to the left, trying to keep the lower body unmoved. Repeat 7 – 9 times.

Lower spinal cord

1. Lock your arms in a crisscross position touching the chest, then sliding locked arms down as far as you can get, holding in that position for a few seconds. Now slowly bend back with arms still locked by the chest, bending the spine as far back as you can (be careful – don't do it too hard), also holding in this position for a few seconds. Repeat 5 – 7 times.

2. Sit down on the chair. Hold your straight hands together in front of you and pull them down at 45 degrees angle towards the floor, bending and stretching your entire spine for 5 seconds. Slowly move your arms up, above and behind you, bending and stretching your spine back for 5 seconds. Repeat 3 – 5 times.

3. Stand straight with legs in a wide but comfortable position. Rest your hands on your hips. Bend your body with the spring motion two times to the left, two times to the right, two times to the front, two times to the back. Repeat the loop 3 – 5 times.

4. Do the same as above, only holding your hands on the back of the head, and instead of four sides do eight sides of a circle. Bend your body with the spring motion two times to each side. Repeat the loop 3 – 5 times.

5. Rest both of your fists on the back just above the waist, putting elbows as close as possible to each other. Push your fists hard into the body, bending the spine at the same time for 5 seconds, then slowly bend your body to the front while still keeping arms behind. Repeat 3 – 5 times.

6. Put your right hand on the back of the head, the left hand behind your back and then bend the body to the left, lifting the right elbow towards the sky. Switch hands and bend the body to the right. Repeat 5 – 7 times.

7. Sit-down with spine and neck straight up, lock your arms in a crisscross position. Turn your head to the side, then shoulders will follow, then the chest, at last the abdomen; try to turn as far as you can, holding that position for 3 seconds. Do the same, turning the other way. Repeat 7 – 9 times.

8. Stand with legs in a wide but comfortable position and place both hands on the back of your head. Turn your entire torso above the waist in a circular motion 5 – 7 full circles in one direction, the same in the other direction. Try to keep bend down as low as possible while doing that. Repeat 3 – 5 times. *This movement, by-the-way, does wonders for those who want to lose weight and build strong stomach and lower spine muscles.*

Lumbar spinal cord

1. Stand with legs in a wide but comfortable position and hold you hands behind your back. Bend your body forward, as far down as you comfortably can, keeping your head up, make 3 – 5 small up-and-down movements while bended down. Do the same bending forward with small angle to the left and to the right.

2. Stand with legs in a wide but comfortable position. While bending back, try to touch your feet with your hands. Repeat 3 – 5 times.

3. Sit down on the floor; legs are straight and slightly spread. Bend your body forward trying to touch the floor with your nose, then bend towards one leg, then towards another leg. Do not over-do it, try to be as relaxed as possible. Repeat 5 – 7 times.

4. Stand with legs in a wide but comfortable position. Bend your body as follows: forward with small up and down movements trying to reach left feet, right feet, then the floor in between with your hands; bend the body back with your hands on the back of your head, stretching as far back as you can. Repeat this 3 – 5 times.

5. Stand with legs in a wide but comfortable position. Hold your right hand up and left hand down, then turn the body to the left,

sliding left hands down trying to reach the feet. Do the same to the opposite side. Repeat 3 – 5 times.

6. While standing with straight legs a slightly wide position, turn your head and upper torso to the left, trying to reach right feet with your left hand. Do the same to the opposite side. Repeat 3 – 5 times.

Don't forget that *all these exercises should be done in relaxed manner*. If you get too tired and did not finish the routine, stop doing this and just walk slowly for a few minutes (do not sit down) and try to relax. Do not try to hurt yourself; you may allow just slight pain when stretching, but not too much. Make this exercise routine as enjoyable as possible. When you finish, you should feel just *slightly* tired.

You should love your body regardless of how it looks, and should treat it with love. There is no other way if you want to see positive results. Never forget the power of your thoughts, and never forget the power of your belief.

Legs and arms workout

1. Stand, spreading your legs wide. Bend your knees, substantially lowering down your body. Keeping legs bended and your body vertical, slowly move the body to the left resting it on the left leg, then to the right resting the body on the right leg. To hold the balance, you may hold. Repeat 15 – 20 times or until you get slightly tired. This movement can also be used as *high-intensity exercise*.

2. Stand, putting your legs together. Bend your knees slightly, holding them together with your hands. Rotate your knees with help of your hands 10 times in one direction, same in the other. Repeat 2 – 3 times.

3. Do sit-ups – fully up and fully down 10 – 15 times or until you get slightly tired. This movement can also be used as *high-intensity exercise*.

4. While standing, make all kinds of movements with your feet, moving the body weight resting point from one spot to another. This exercise ideally should be performed barefooted. Do this for 1 minute.

5. Rise up on your toes and lower yourself down, walk on your toes. This ideally should be performed barefooted. **Attention**: this exercise is very important not only because it stimulates feet joints and growth plates, but also because it *stimulates the release of growth hormone*. It happens because there is a small area near the center of the pad of the big toe (called "pituitary gland reflex area") that if stimulated, it affects the work of the pituitary gland that is responsible for the production and release of growth hormone into the body. Massaging that spot is also very helpful, and we have already discussed how to do it correctly in the section "Stimulating Reflex Zones" of the chapter "Human Growth Hormone".

6. Stand-up. While trying to keep your arm relaxed, rotate it forward along with a shoulder moderately fast 10 – 15 rotations, constantly changing the angle of the rotation, then the same backwards. Do the same with another arm. Repeat 3 – 5 times.

7. Stand-up. With both of your arms parallel to the floor, move them simultaneously with fast motion far back, then crossing them in the front, while slowly turning your body to the right and to the left. Do 15 – 25 arm movements.

Chin-up bar workout

The chin-up bar should be your great companion for as long as you are working on increasing your height, and hopefully long after. Any time you have a moment to hang on the bar, just do it. There are an endless number of exercises you can do on the chin-up bar, however some of them could cause injuries unless you are an expert at gymnastics. *All you need to do in the scope of this program is hang, trying to keep your body relaxed, even if it is difficult to relax when you start.*

For some people it might be hard to hold onto the bar; their hands might not be strong enough. If you are one of those people you should push yourself to do it anyway, and each time you go on the bar, it will become easier to hold yourself up than it was the time before, because your hands will be getting stronger.

Here are some other ways to make your hands stronger and be ready for the chin-up bar workout:

- Tighten your fists hard and rotate them until your arm muscles feel tired.

- Use a rubber or spring hand flexor (which can be found in any sports equipment store).

- Hold 2 – 3 lbs (1 – 1.3 kg) dumbbells in your hands and rotate your wrists like a propeller back and forth, holding your arms in any position, but not moving them

---

I strongly advise you to have a chin-up bar in your home. This should be your only exercise equipment. It is a special bar made for home use that can be installed between two vertical surfaces (walls) that are close to each other, or on the doorframe. It must be high enough so your feet should not touch the floor when you hang from the bar. Don't forget – you will be growing taller, and one day you may be too tall for the height of the bar. The distance from your feet to the floor when hanging should be at least 4 – 7 inches. *You are probably thinking that 7 or even 4 inches of height gains are impossible.* Think again. ***Make it your goal, do your best, and one day your friends might not recognize you.*** You can buy this type of bar at your local sports equipment store or online. Go to www.grow-taller.com/bar for suggestions and links to where it is sold.

When you purchase the chin-up bar, try to find the type that is not slippery because the less slippery it is – the longer you will be able to hang-on. The best are those that have comfortable foam grips. If you already have one that is slippery, to make it less slippery wrap the chin-up bar with one layer of masking tape.

When you feel more comfortable hanging from the bar, the way to relax on it is also important: Imagine yourself as just a peace of rope hanging, with no muscles and no bones. Got the picture? Now try to feel some mass of energy inside your chest (it is there) and imagine that this mass of energy is slowly moving down through your body toward your legs, then through your legs toward your feet, and then out of your body. And that is what will actually happen. *This way the stressful energy that you have will leave your body while automatically being replaced with new fresh energy coming from the surroundings, helping you to relax.* Follow these suggestions:

◆ Rotate your body 90 degrees to the right and 90 degrees to the left. Use your arms to move the body. This is easy to do and effective.

◆ Imagine that you are riding a bicycle and rotating invisible bicycle pedals. Your body and legs should be relaxed and rotating should be spontaneous. This exercise will give a good push for your leg's growth.

◆ Push your legs as far as possible from each other in any direction, to the front and the back or to the sides, switching leg positions back and forth.

◆ Shake your body using small wrist flexes up and down with your hands still on the bar. Your body should be "loose as a lifeless rope".

♦ Relax for the first few seconds then lift your legs up, bending them at your knees, as high as possible. Keep this position for 20 – 30 seconds, then slowly lower down your legs and release the bar. Rest for 1 – 2 minutes, and then repeat this exercise one more time.

I recommend doing chin-ups, especially for men. This will not only give you stronger arms, neck, shoulders, and chest muscles, but is a great way to perform *high-intensity exercise* (do as many chin-ups in one series as you can) that helps to **increase the release of growth hormone**. Often change hands positions (changing distance between hands, facing hands forward, backwards). This way you will involve most muscles of your upper body.

> There is no limit on how many times and for how long you can hang on the bar. The more you do it – the better.

One of the best bar exercises you can do is on monkey bars that are built in many parks and playgrounds, which look like an extension ladder that was laid out horizontally. It should be high enough from the ground for you not to touch it with your legs while hanging from it. All you need is just to move under it with hands: hang on the first bar, then grab the next bar with one hand, remove another hand a second later, moving it to the next bar and so on and on. When you feel comfortable enough doing this (after some practice), you can try skipping one or even two bars, reaching for the third one.

This exercise may be a little tough in the beginning, even causing calluses on your hands, but this is **one of the best exercises you can do to help your body grow** because it will involve and stimulate most bone growth plates in your body and most muscles, stretching them at the same time. Monkey bars are also great for any other bar exercises that were mentioned above.

If you have never tried monkey bar or rarely did it, please be careful and do not over-do-it in the beginning because this way your hands will quickly get callus formation that can easily be ripped. Callus formation building up on the skin is actually what you need because gripping the bar remains painful as long as you don't have calluses. *The trick here is to gradually increase using monkey bar, slowly toughen-up the skin with calluses.* In addition, to avoid callus formation you should grip the bar carefully, trying not to fold your skin.

If you got ripped calluses, here's what you can do: Cut the ripped skin away using scissors, disinfect, and wrap nose tissue around your hand when working out.

It will take up to 2 weeks for your hand to heal. Count another 2 weeks for your skin to toughen up. During those 2 weeks you can rip of the calluses again. So make sure you grip the bar correctly.

Jumps

Jumps are extremely helpful in your quest to increase your height. When you make jumps, there are many things happen that boost your growth:

◆ You unintentionally lengthen your energy twin, which automatically lengthen the body (see "The Power Of Mind" section of this book above). The way it works – when we jump trying to reach high placed object, we are not only stretching our body, we are imagining our body stretching. That imagination, that thought, is what makes the energy twin to stretch, forcing the body to grow.

◆ You stretch all your muscles, reducing resistance of your body to grow.

◆ Practically all bone growth plates and spinal disks in the body are well stimulated.

◆ You increase and normalize circulation of blood reach of oxygen in the body, stimulating the process of your body's development and growth.

◆ The small area near the center of the pad of the big toe (called "pituitary gland reflex area") is well stimulated while we jump, in turn – ***stimulating the release of growth hormone.*** We have already discussed this reflex area in the "Legs and arms workout" section this chapter, and you already know how it works.

Why do you think all professional basketball players are taller than anybody else? Yes, because they jump a lot. All of them spent big portion of their childhood and early adulthood constantly jumping, trying to reach high placed object (basket). Please understand, *they are playing basketball not because they are tall,* ***they are tall because they are playing basketball.*** You don't have to play basketball to achieve great results, just follow these suggestions:

1. Jump with both of your feet from the same spot trying to reach some high overhanging object (like branch of a tree). Do 7 – 9 jumps, then bend your knees and your body down for a few seconds, and then jump again. Repeat 2 – 3 times. Do these jumps with all your power, jumping as high as possible. Do not rush, and if you get tired – have some intervals between jumps. Rest afterward by walking slowly for 2 – 3 minutes.

2. Jump in the same spot while trying to reach the same object, only this time using one leg at a time: 10 times from the left leg, relax for 20 seconds; 10 times from the right leg, relax for 20 seconds; 10 times hopping from one leg to the other, switching each time (30 jumps altogether). Rest afterward by walking slowly for 3 – 5 minutes.

3. Do the reaching jumps with a running start. Start about 12 – 15 feet (4 – 5 meters) from the object you want to reach. Run slowly toward this object, making the last two steps faster, then jump while pushing up with both of your feet and stretching your body

out to touch the object with your both hands. Basically, this is the same type of jump as used in basketball to reach the basket. Do these leaps 5 times, then, after a short break, repeat them 10 times switching legs from which to jump.

I do not recommend doing jumps less than one hour before or after meals or less than two hours before sleep. All other times, use any convenient moment to do jumps: at home or school – reaching for the ceiling, outside – reaching for the branches of trees or any other objects.

You need to do 200 – 300 jumps every day. If you do more, it will not hurt. As was mentioned above, playing basketball is the best way to reach your jumps quantity goal. Volleyball is also great, as well as any other sport game that has these types of jumps.

Suggestions for outdoors exercises

The best place for exercises, especially in the morning, is outdoors. All exercises mentioned in this book can be performed outside. Even though most of our exercise activities can also be performed at home, in a gym or a fitness club, nothing will replace sun and fresh air (see "Affects of Sun" chapter in this book).

Suggestions for exercises at home

If you do exercises at home, first make sure you have enough room in your house, no neighbors will be disturbed and no furniture is on your way. Here is what you will need:

Open the window. *You need fresh air, and your body needs oxygen.* The indoor exercise program is almost the same as the outdoor program. The difference is that you might not have enough room for running and some jumps, unless you have a home gym with a track for running, or you do this workout at your local fitness center.

If you don't have enough room for some of exercises, here is an alternative:

While warming-up, you can skip the slow run and do light, relaxing jumps instead. A treadmill would be a great piece of exercise equipment to own because *slow* running is the most powerful exercise for improving and keeping your health in good shape, however you can do just well without it.

Running is just a good way to prepare yourself for the main exercise. You can also replace distance running with running in place (continuous light jogging, keeping both legs pumping). An indoor object that can be used in this program instead of the tree branch is any high overhanging object that you can only reach by jumping, such as a ceiling or a cloth placed high enough so that it is hard for you to reach.

Additional exercises

These exercises *may not be included* in the routine, however all of them may affect your body's development and growth.

1. Lay flat on your back, bringing both knees to your chest. From this position, wrap your arms around your legs pushing your knees closer to the chest, while trying to reach your chest with your chin. Hold this position for 15 – 20 seconds. Repeat 2 – 3 times.

2. Lay flat on your back, knees bent, and feet flat on the floor. Let both legs fall to one side, then to the other side. Each time hold for 10 seconds.

3. Hands and knees on the floor: stay on all fours, resting most of your weight on your knees. Then move your body toward your hands, do one push-up, then move back as far as you can, trying to sit on your feet, then get back to the push-up, over and over again 15 – 20 times. Your hands should stay in the same spot all the time.

4. Push-ups are not only another great way to strengthen your arms, chest, and back muscles. They strengthen the heart, filling the bloodstream with oxygen and growth hormone. You can work on different muscles placing your hands at different distances from each other and at different angles. This exercise can be used as *high-intensity exercise.*

5. Lay flat on your back, arms fully extended over your head, legs fully extended on the floor; extend your whole body from your fingertips to your toes, lengthening your body in both directions. While in this posture, turn your upper body to the left and to the right while keeping your hips on the floor. This exercise is also great while you are in bed.

If you are tired and your heart is beating fast, the technique below is very practical to reduce your heartbeat and get a lot of extra energy for your body:

Walk slowly for a while. Spread both arms horizontally in one line, with your palms facing up so you look like a cross. Imagine a lot of pure energy around your body. Breathe the air in, while slowly moving both arms up and then down, crossing each other in front of you while letting the air out. While doing this, imagine grabbing pure and powerful energy from outside, and inserting it into your body. Do this a few times, until your heartbeat has decreased and you feel rested.

Your posture

If you want to maximize your growth, ***the way you sit, the way you stand, and the way you walk are very important***. Right now, while reading this, pay attention to your posture. Is your neck bent down a little, trying to hold your heavy head, or are you are holding your head straight up? How about your spine? Is it straight or does it look like a question mark? Yes, this is important for your body. Spinal disks should have as little pressure as possible, and the way to minimize that pressure *you should keep your back straight at all times.*

Imagine your body growing right now really quickly while slowly stretching your entire body up as high as possible, making it look and feel like you are growing about one inch (2 – 3 cm) in just a few seconds. Stay in this position for a few seconds then relax while keeping the same pose. *This is the posture you should keep for the rest of your life.* ***This will not only make it easier for your body to grow, this position of the body will prevent many diseases in the future, it will be harder for you to get tired, even your brain will work better.***

Another way to find the right posture for your body is to stay against the wall touching the wall with your back, shoulders and head. Spread your shoulders wider, but not too much, to be comfortable.

When you are holding an object in your hands, especially when it is heavy, try to keep is as close to the body as possible, to minimize the pressure on the spine. The best way to carry something is to use the backpack.

Very soft mattress you sleep on may also bring negative affect to your posture, so a firmer mattress is a must.

During the course of the day, no matter what you do, stretch your body up as described above at any convenient moment. *Stretching by itself does not make the body grow, but it creates the good "foundation" to make the most out of your growth potentials.* Force your body to grow and do it right.

If You Are a Bodybuilder or Weightlifter

[skeleton]

It is perfectly acceptable to have strong muscles, but huge muscles are not necessarily good for your health (often not) and may actually affect your body's height. This happens because when muscles are too stiff, they keep entire skeleton under constant pressure, even at night. It does not necessarily mean however that you should quit. You may actually continue without side effects, even benefiting your body's growth from this activity if you follow my advices.

Principals of safe weightlifting are simple:

◆ Do not over-do it. Too much stress will stiffen-up your muscles, may make them bigger, but not necessarily stronger. It will put your entire body under constant pressure even when you are not performing the work-out, preventing it from growing taller. Too much stress is very damaging to the heart and entire body. I also recommend doing all muscle exercises at a slower pace.

◆ Try to keep your muscles as relaxed as possible. Constantly massage every muscle you are working on, constantly stretch them, often jump or shake your body, hang on the chin-up bar in between exercises.

◆ Do not put a lot of stress on your spine, so avoid lifting heavy objects in a stand-up position. Try to do most weight-lifting in lay-down position.

◆ Mix weightlifting with exercises recommended in this book (see above) at the same time.

◆ Do not take any steroids or other chemicals to enhance your muscles. This will hurt you in the long run.

A good practice to build strong muscles is by holding the muscles under pressure without moving them. All movements should be made in between, for the purpose of relaxation. This way your muscles may not be as large, but they will definitely be stronger than larger muscles, at the same time – more flexible.

There is one thing with which *weightlifting can actually help you to boost your body's growth*. As it was previously mentioned in the book, resistance or high-intensity exercise (physical stress during a relatively short period of time) can be incredibly effective at increasing growth hormone level in the blood, released by the pituitary gland. Weightlifting is one of good options to perform resistance or high-intensity exercise. Pick the maximum weight you can lift that you will be able to hold up to 30 seconds, pick it up and hold it until you cannot hold it anymore. Just keep in mind that you should do it no more than once or twice for around 30 seconds but no more than 60 seconds at each instance. Second time should be not earlier than 1 hour after the first time. I do not recommend performing this stress exercise more often than 3 times a day. Also, prepare yourself with regular exercise for at least several minutes that involve the same muscles that you are planning to use in this high-intensity exercise.

Swimming

A swimming pool should be your best "fitness room". There is no better exercise for most parts of your body than swimming. When we are in the water, gravitation does not affect our body, as it does when you are on the ground. This means that nothing stops your body from growing while you swim. Have you ever noticed how tall swimmers are?

It is not necessary for you to swim very fast, or to learn special swimming techniques. All you will need is just to be able to stay afloat and do only one swimming technique: *the basic breaststroke*. This requires strokes of your legs and arms at the same time, essentially stretching your entire boy each time you take a stroke. Three – four times a week of one-hour swim will give your body's development a great boost.

As we discussed in the chapter "Breathing", swimming under water is a very powerful technique to boost your growth hormone level. To do that, you basically do the same breaststroke swimming technique, just diving under water *close to the surface* for as long as you can hold (don't overexert yourself). Before diving-in, exhale as much of the air in your lungs as possible, and then inhale as much as possible, do it again and then dive. When diving, try to be very calm, concentrate on the time or distance spent underwater. Just be careful not to swallow any water.

As great as swimming is, if you don't have a swimming pool or a beach near you or simply cannot afford it, don't be discouraged. Following the exercise program described in this book will be enough for you to reach maximum of your growth potential, without swimming. Nevertheless, use every opportunity to swim, especially in the sea or the ocean (*salt water is great for our health*).

What to Eat

What do we need to eat? What type of diet do we need to follow? I want you to know right from the beginning – I don't agree with the "eating too much or too little" theories or diets. My stand on this is: **what you eat and when you eat is more important than how much you eat.** *You should eat as much as you are comfortable with.* Some people may say – well, what if a person is comfortable eating too much? The trick is – if you follow my recommendations in this book, especially exercise and water intake, your body will function properly, and will regulate the amount of food you will want to take. You simply will not want to eat more than your body needs. Even when sometimes you overeat – your body will deal with that easily. Once again, it will be that way only if you follow my recommendations.

Just so you know, *obesity does reduce the production of growth hormone.* It was proven by several scientific groups. This should be another reason for you to eat right and follow other advises in this book.

As we learned earlier in the "Dieting Strategies" section of "Growth Hormone" paragraph, one of the biggest contributors for the release of growth hormone is the right food. The growth hormone production triggered by food intake depends on:

- Level of carbohydrates in food we consume
- The amount of insulin those carbohydrates help to produce
- Amino acids contained in some foods
- The amount of fat in foods
- Timing of food intake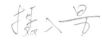

Keep in mind that as much as we need growth hormone to increase the body's height, eating the right food in our program is not only designed to boost your growth hormone level, but it is designed to keep your body functioning properly.

> *Everything in our body is connected on many levels including physical and energy level. That is why we should not concentrate only on one particular function; we should concentrate on the entire body as a whole. Only that will bring us ultimate results.*

Before I will describe what to eat, I want you to understand the process of growth hormone release triggered by food.

After every meal our bodies go through a three-stage cycle:

1. In the first hour after eating, the blood sugar rises and insulin (a hormone responsible for the metabolism of sugar) is released, which supports the storage of excess carbohydrates and fat.

2. After the second hour, release of growth hormone begins and the level of insulin and blood sugar starts to fall. Growth hormone acts to build up muscle and bone protein, with help of insulin.

3. Four hours or more after eating, the growth hormone concentrations are still at the high level, while insulin almost disappears. At this stage, growth hormone is breaking down the body's fat, using it as fuel to create energy.

If the growth hormone level remains low, insulin is free to turn almost every calorie into fat for later use. That is why we are gaining fat! If the insulin level remains low, growth hormone can melt away fat, which is our energy storage. Insulin, growth hormone and fat are our friends, and the balance between them is very important. So, how can we keep this balance? Simple! Your body will create this balance if you follow my recommendations in food intake and everything else in our program you have already learned.

Your body needs nutrients (chemical elements that make up a food) to function properly and to maintain the right level of growth hormone and other important hormones. The nutrients we all need include **carbohydrates**, **proteins**, **fats**, **vitamins**, and **minerals**. Your body gets these nutrients from the foods you eat. Nutrients give your body what you need for metabolism, which is set of chemical reactions in the body that convert the fuel from food into the energy needed to do everything from moving to thinking to growing.

Carbohydrates

Carbohydrates are the fuel for our body. They are the primary energy source for all our activities. They are found in almost all foods that we eat.

When carbohydrates get into our body, they are being broken down and used as energy. When the body doesn't need to use the carbohydrates for energy, it stores them into the liver and muscles in form of "glycogen". When the liver and muscles cells cannot store anymore glycogen, it is turned into fat. When your body needs a quick boost of energy, it converts glycogen into energy. When it needs a prolonged burst of energy, it converts fat to energy.

As you understand the importance of carbohydrates, let me bring-out one very important fact: *food that contains carbohydrates can* ***decrease*** *the release of growth hormone, even completely stop it*. That is why it is very important for you to read and understand the following.

Carbohydrates contain sugars that are easily dissolved in the blood, raising its sugar concentration. When this concentration is too high (high blood sugar), it directly affects the production of the growth hormone.

Does it mean we should avoid eating foods that contain carbohydrates? Absolutely not. We need carbohydrates for the energy, moreover, carbohydrates trigger the release of insulin which promotes the benefits of growth hormone; we just need to control how much sugars are dissolved in our blood. Sounds complicated, but it is not. The trick is – different carbohydrate foods (carbs) dissolve sugars into blood differently, some faster, some slower. If we will eat mostly carbohydrate foods that dissolve its sugars slowly, the level of our blood sugar will be normal, and the growth hormone release will flow as it should (also depending on other factors described in this book).

How do we know which carbs dissolve its sugars slower and which faster? Scientists have created a scale called "glycemic index" that measures how fast carbohydrates are absorbed into the bloodstream and how long it takes to raise the blood sugar level. This glycemic index shows the number next to each type of food. The higher the number – the higher glycemic index, the lower the number – the lower glycemic index. See glycemic index table on the next page.

If you consume large amount of high glycemic carbs, you could completely halt growth hormone release. Or more generally speaking – a high carbohydrate and low fat diet is absolutely devastating to growth hormone levels. This is one of the reasons why many people unsuccessfully trying to lose weight on such a diet. Their inability to continue to lose weight is partly due to suppressed growth hormone levels.

> *Eating a lot of foods that rank high on the glycemic index not only affects our body's growth, but also may lead us to obesity.*

We will arrive to the conclusion with understanding that *an ideal growth hormone enhancing diet should include some carbs, but not an excessive amount.* And the focus should be on carbs with **low** glycemic index.

Table on the next page is a very important and powerful tool that will help you to chose what to eat and in what amounts. As you will learn later in this chapter, most recommendations on food intake fall along guidelines of this table. That is why you should first brefly look at this table, then read explanations on following pages, then go back and examine the table closely. You will need to use it, preferably for your entire life if you want to be not only taller, but much healthier.

Keep in mind: *Carbohydrates should be about **50-65%** of your daily consumption*

Glycemic Index / Glycemic Load

Type	GI	SS	GL
Fruit			
Apple	38	120	6
Apricots	36	120	3
Apricots, dried	35	60	7
Banana	56	120	13
Blueberries, wild	53	100	5
Cantaloupe	65	120	4
Cherries	23	120	3
Dates	103	60	42
Figs, dried	61	60	16
Grapefruit	26	120	3
Grapes	46	120	8
Kiwi	52	120	6
Mango	56	120	9
Orange	43	120	4
Papaya	58	120	10
Peach	42	120	5
Pear	37	120	4
Pineapple	66	120	7
Plantain	38	120	13
Plums	39	120	5
Prunes	29	60	10
Raisins	64	60	28
Raspberry	27	25	3
Strawberries	32	120	1
Watermelon	72	120	4
Breakfast Cereals			
All Bran	51	30	9
Bran Buds + psyll	47	30	6
Bran Flakes	74	30	13
Cheerios	74	30	15
Corn Chex	83	30	21
Cornflakes	77	30	20
Corn Pops	80	30	21
Cream of Wheat	66	250	17
Frosted Flakes	55	30	18
Grapenuts	71	30	15
Just right	66	30	14
Komplete	48	30	10
Muesli, natural	54	30	10
Nutri-grain	66	30	10
Oatmeal, old fash	40	250	30

Type	GI	SS	GL
Pop Tarts	70	50	25
Puffed Wheat	80	30	17
Raisin Bran	73	30	14
Rice Chex	89	30	23
Rice krispies	82	30	22
Shredded Wheat	70	30	14
Special K	54	30	11
Total	76	30	17
Nuts			
Almonds	0	50	0
Brazil Nuts	0	50	0
Cashew Nuts	22	50	3
Hazelnuts	0	50	0
Macadamia Nuts	0	50	0
Peanuts	14	50	1
Pecan Nuts	0	50	0
Walnuts	0	50	0
Snacks & Sweets			
Chocolate, Dark (70%)	22	50	6
Chocolate, Milk, Plain	43	50	12
Croissant	67	57	17
Corn chips	72	50	11
Doughnut	76	47	17
French fries	75	150	22
Graham Wafers	74	25	14
Ice cream, 2 scoops	61	50	8
Jelly beans	80	30	22
Life Savers	70	30	21
Marmalade	48	30	9
Mars bar	62	60	25
M & M	68	60	27
Oatmeal cookie	54	25	9
Kudos Whole-Grain Bars	62	50	20
Potato chips	56	50	11
Pound cake	54	53	15
Power bar	56	65	24
Pretzels	83	30	16
Rice cakes	80	25	17

Type	GI	SS	GL
Saltine crackers	74	25	13
Shortbread cookies	64	25	8
Snickers bar	68	60	23
Sponge cake	45	63	17
Strawberry jam	51	30	10
Tofu frozen dessert	115	50	10
Twix cookie bar	44	60	17
Vanilla wafers	77	25	14
Water cracker	71	25	13
Wheat Thins	67	25	12
Pasta			
Cheese tortellini	50	180	10
Fettucini	32	180	18
Instant noodles	47	180	19
Linguini	50	180	23
Macaroni	46	180	23
Refined pasta	65	180	26
Rice pasta	92	180	35
Spaghetti, 15 min boiled	58	180	28
Spaghetti, 5 min boiled	33	180	16
Spaghetti, protein enrich	28	180	14
Vermicelli	35	180	16
Whole grain pasta	45	180	20
Beverages			
Apple juice	40	250	12
Coca Cola	65	250	16
Cranberry juice	52	250	16
Fanta	68	250	23
Gatorade	78	250	12
Grapefruit juice	48	250	9
Lucozade	95	250	40
Orange juice	46	250	12
Pineapple juice	48	250	15
Smoothie, raspberry	33	250	14
Smoothie, soy	30	250	7
Tomato juice	37	250	4

Type	GI	SS	GL	Type	GI	SS	GL	Type	GI	SS	GL
Vegetables				Long Grain Rice	60	150	25	Croissant	67	57	17
Artichokes	0	80	0	Millet	71	150	25	Dark rye	76	30	10
Avocado	0	80	0	Popcorn	72	20	8	Hamburger bun	61	30	9
Beets	64	80	5	Puffed rice	95	150	40	Muffin apple cinnamon	44	60	13
Broccoli	0	80	0	Quick Cook Rice	65	150	28	Oat & raisin	54	50	14
Cabbage	0	80	0	Taco shells	68	20	8	Oat bran bread	47	30	9
Carrots	16	80	1	White rice	70	150	30	Pita	57	30	10
Carrots, boiled	38	80	2	Whole grain rye	34	50	13	Pizza plain	80	100	22
Cauliflower	0	80	0					Pizza, cheese	60	100	16
Celery	0	80	0	**Sweeteners**				Pumpernickel	49	30	5
Chickpeas	36	150	11	Agave nectar	11	10	1	Rye bread	50	30	6
Corn sweet	54	80	9	Corn syrup	62	10	11	Sourdough	54	30	6
Cucumber	0	80	0	Fructose	20	10	2	Whole wheat bread	70	30	13
Green peas	51	80	3	Glucose	100	10	10				
Instant potatoes	85	150	17	Honey	62	25	11	White bread	70	30	10
Lettuce	0	80	0	Maltodextrin	105	10	12	Whole grain bread	59	30	7
Parsnips	97	80	12	Maltose	105	10	11	Pastry	59	60	15
Peppers	0	80	0	Stevia	0	5	0				
Potatoes sweet	50	150	17	Table sugar	65	10	7	**Milk Products**			
Potatoes baked	85	150	26					Chocolate milk	35	250	9
Potatoes boiled	58	150	16	**Beans**				Cheese	0	120	0
Potatoes mashed	74	150	15	Baked beans	44	150	7	Custard	43	100	7
Potatoes microwaved	82	150	27	Black beans, boiled	30	150	7	Ice cream, vanilla	61	50	8
Pumpkin	75	80	3	Butter beans, boiled	33	150	6	Ice cream, chocolate	68	50	9
Rutabaga	71	150	7	Cannellini beans	31	150	6	Ice milk, vanilla	50	250	6
Spinach	0	80	0	French beans	0	80	0	Milk, fat free	32	250	4
Squash	0	80	0	Garbanzo, boiled	34	150	8	Milk, full fat	27	250	3
Tomatoes	38	150	2	Kidney, boiled	23	150	6	Mousse	34	50	4
Yam	66	150	13	Kidney, canned	52	150	9	Soy milk	30	250	8
Onion	10	80	5	Lentils, green, brown	30	150	6	Soy Smoothie Drink	30	250	7
Mushroom				Lentils, red, boiled	21	150	4	Skim milk	32	250	4
				Lima beans, boiled	32	150	10	Whole milk	30	250	3
Grains & Rice				Navy beans	31	150	9	Yogurt, fruit	38	200	11
Arborio rice	69	150	36	Pinto, boiled	39	150	10	Yogurt, plain	36	200	3
Barley	25	150	26	Soybeans, boiled	16	150	1				
Basmati white rice	58	150	22					**Meats & fish**			
Brown rice	55	150	18	**Breads**				All fresh meats and fish	0	-	0
Buckwheat	45	150	13	Bagel, plain	72	70	25				
Bulgur wheat	48	150	12	Baguette, French	95	30	14	Eggs	0	120	0
Corn tortilla	52	50	12	Blueberry muffin	59	70	22	Sausages	28	100	1
Cornmeal	68	150	9	Bran muffin	52	70	17				
Couscous	65	150	23								
Instant rice	87	150	36								

*GI – *Glycemic Index*   **SS** – *Serving Size (in grams and mL)*   **GL** – *Glycemic Load*

The glycemic index uses glucose as the baseline with its index set as being equal to 100.

If you did not find some food that you usually eat is this list, go to *www.grow-taller.com/gi_gl* for a complete International list of glycemic index (GI) and glycemic load (GL) values published by The American Journal of Clinical Nutrition.

To easily figure-out the serving size, follow this reference:

- 30 grams = 1 oz (ounce) = 1/8 cup
- 60 grams = 2 oz = 1/4 cup = 1/8 lb (pound)
- 110 grams = 4 oz = 1/2 cup = 1/4 lb
- 225 grams = 8 oz = 1 cup = 1/2 lb

You should understand that glycemic index value for each food is not precise, and may vary depending on many factors such as method of preparation, growing conditions, geographic locations, genetic strain, acidity, food particle size (smaller particles are absorbed faster), ripeness, fiber, protein and fat content of this food, as well as accompanying foods (fat and protein decrease the speed with which the stomach empties, thus decreasing the rate of carbohydrate absorption, reducing food's glycemic index).

In addition, the impact a food will have on your blood sugar level depends on time of the day you take this food, your blood insulin levels, your recent physical activities, as well as content and timing of the previous meal. In general, the index value may fluctuate in the range of ± 3 to 8. Also, if you mix or simultaneously eat different foods, the glycemic index value will be the average index of all these foods combined. For example, if you eat cornflakes cereal (77) with whole milk (30), the average glycemic index value of this meal will be approximately 53.

Another important factor you should understand is that each food listed in the glycemic index table has different percentage of carbohydrates in it. For example, 120 grams of watermelon does not mean 120 grams of carbohydrates, but only 6 grams, as watermelons has very low percentile of carbohydrates in them. Therefore, when deciding on what food to eat, you need to look at much more important value called **glycemic load**, which is *calculated by multiplying the glycemic index by the amount of carbohydrate in grams in food and dividing the total by 100.* You don't have to remember this formula, just look at already calculated numbers at **Glycemic Index / Glycemic Load** table above, however most prepackaged foods have the size of the serving and the amount of carbohydrates per serving in grams shown on the packaging.

Use amount of carbohydrates shown on the packaging, multiplying it by glycemic index and dividing by 100 to get the most precise glycemic load value for this prepackaged food.

> To make it simple, this **Glycemic Index / Glycemic Load** table displays *Glycemic Index, Serving Size,* and *Glycemic Load per serving size.* By using this table as the reference, you will know exactly what to eat without blocking the release of growth hormone. Moreover, by following Glycemic index suggestions to increase growth hormone level, you will also benefit tremendously with your general health, which is also extremely important for your growth. Remember the phrase – "you are what you eat"? This is true because *if you are not treating your body well by eating the good food, your body will eventually suffer* and will even affect your spirit.

By the way, what is described here can apply to a person of any age, so if you care about health of your older ones, tell them that this diet can give better benefits for general health and loosing weight than any other diet.

Lets look at what is considered *low, medium* and *high* values of glycemic index and glycemic load:

Glycemic Index (GI)	Glycemic Load (GL)
Low – 0 to 55	Low – 0 to 10
Medium – 56 to 70	Medium – 11 to 19
High – 71 to 100	High – 20 and more

Foods that have a low GL almost always have a low GI. Foods with medium or high GL range from very low to very high GI. Also, most (but not all) foods with high GI are highly processed carbohydrates with very little fiber and few nutrients.

After all, what should I eat, what I should not eat, and in what amounts? – you will ask. As the general rule, majority of the food that we eat should have *low* and *medium* value of glycemic index, and the maximum daily amount of carbs you should consume can be easily measured by glycemic load and calculated by this formula:

Total maximum daily glycemic load =	your weight in pounds / 1.3
	your weight in kilograms / 0.6

Your **minimum** daily glycemic load could be 30 less in value.

As an example, if your body weight is 120 pounds – your maximum glycemic load per day should be 120 / 1.3 = 92, or it should be between 62 and 92.

Also keep in mind that this formula is good only if you are performing exercise routine described in this book. If you don't exercise (which I don't recommend), you should *decrease* your maximum daily glycemic load value by about 30%. If you are in sports, and performing much more intensive physical activities than what is recommended in this book, you should *increase* your maximum daily glycemic load value by 20 – 50% depending on how intensive your sport is.

Glycemic load is the fuel or the energy that your body receives from food, and the more energy you use, the higher your daily glycemic load value should be. For those who sometimes do extreme physical activities (I hope you are not one of those), it is even a good idea to give a "boost" to the "power supply" by consuming more carbs with higher glycemic load value – right before these activities.

How do you breakdown the amounts of all foods that you should eat? Just calculate in advance. Usually it is convenient to make a plan for the next day, even better for the entire week. Select what you would like to eat, figure approximately the weight of each dish, and then check with the glycemic index table shown above to calculate the total glycemic load value of each dish. Add glycemic load values of all dishes and snacks you are planning to eat in one day and see if the total number is within your limits. If not, try to redesign the food combination to fit into your limits. It may sound complicated, but it is not; after the first time you try, it will become clear to you. In a very short period of time of such food planning, you will know exactly what you need to eat and in what amounts, without making many more calculations.

If all of the above is too complicated for you, lets simplify by describing general suggestions on what carbs you should eat and what you should try to avoid:

Eat more:

♦ Most of the vegetables (except potato) including alfalfa, asparagus, beans, broccoli, cabbage, carrots, cauliflower, chickpeas, cucumber, garlic, green beans, kale, kidney beans, leek, lentils, lettuce, mushrooms, onion, peas, pepper, radishes, soybean, spinach, squash, tomatoes, zucchini.

♦ Almost all the fruits including Apple, banana, blueberry,

cherries, grapefruit, green grapes, kiwi, oranges, peaches, pears, plums, prunes, raspberry, strawberries.

◆ Nuts such as almonds, brazils, macadamias, peanuts, pine nuts, and walnuts.

◆ Seeds such as hemp, linseeds/flax, pumpkin, sesame, and sunflower.

◆ Pulses such as dried beans, chickpeas, and lentils

◆ High fiber, whole grain bread

◆ Plain yogurt

◆ High fiber, unsweetened cereals such as All Bran and muesli

◆ Sweet potatoes

◆ Brown basmati rice, buckwheat grains, quinoa, bulgur wheat, pearl barley

◆ Whole-wheat pasta

Eat less:

◆ Ripe bananas

◆ Fruit yogurts and desserts high in sugar such as imitation mousse

◆ Dried figs, dates

◆ Sweet pies

◆ Fruit canned in syrup

- Breakfast cereals containing sugar

- Rice, especially white rice

- Pasta and spaghetti

- Pizza

- Thickened soups

Severely restrict

- White bread, baguettes, bagels

- Sweets/sugar candy and chocolate bars/chocolate candy

- Cream crackers, white rice cakes

- Iced cakes and pastries, filled biscuits/cookies, doughnuts

- Scones, crumpets, waffles

- Baked and mashed potatoes, chips/fries

- Table sugar

- High sugar jams/jelly

- Fruit drinks containing added sugar

- Ice cream containing glucose syrup or high levels of other sugars

- Fizzy drinks containing sugar

- Crisps/chips and other potato- and corn-based snacks

- Canned spaghetti

If you really like sweets, this may hurt to know that eating too much of candy and other sweets may actually stunt you growth. *If you are seriously thinking to increase your height, you should seriously think to control the amounts of sweets that you eat, and, of cause, follow all my other recommendations.*

Additional suggestions:

- ◆ Choose whole-grain foods over highly processed ones.

- ◆ Packaged/processed cereals can be replaced by homemade or raw muesli made from oats, bran, seeds, and psyllium with small amounts of dried fruit or barley or oats (not instant).

- ◆ To lower the GI of foods, you can add lemon juice, olive oil, flax seed oil, and vinegar. It will slow the absorption of carbohydrates when eaten.

- ◆ To counteract a meal's high GI, eat a green salad with acidic dressing.

- ◆ Add several different types of vegetables to dishes to slow carbohydrate absorption. *Adding two or three times more vegetables than meat or fish can be an easy way to balance the meal.*

- ◆ Choose fruit juices over sugary soft drinks.

- ◆ Replace white bread or bagels with whole grain, pumpernickel or stone-ground wheat breads.

- ◆ Replace white or wheat flour cracker with stone ground or vita-wheat crackers.

- ◆ Instead of sugar use xylitol or stevia – safe natural sweeteners.

- ◆ Replace baked potato with basmati rice, wholegrain rice or sweet potato.

◆ Replace regular milk chocolate with dark chocolate.

◆ Replace white rice with basmati rice or wholegrain rice.

◆ Replace biscuits and cookies with small handful of nuts, or raw vegetable sticks with cheese.

◆ Replace all sodas with plain water (see chapter "Water" in this book).

◆ Replace all sweets and candies with fresh and dry fruits and nuts.

Please understand that individual foods cannot be considered "good" or "bad." It's *how you build your meals* and structure your overall eating plan that counts. For example, if you eat a high GI food (like a baked potato) with protein (like grilled chicken), fiber, and fat (like a spinach salad with an oil-based dressing), the overall glycemic effect of the meal is much lower. Protein, fiber, and fat all slowing digestion and delaying blood sugar release, creating good conditions for the release of growth hormone.

Let me give you a simple example that will highlight the truthfulness of all that is stated here. If you looked at glycemic index table above, have you noticed that rice has one of the highest glycemic loads? It means that theoretically, people who consume a lot of rice on the daily basis throughout their lives should be shorter than others who consume much smaller amounts of carbohydrates. Understanding this, I decided to find a confirmation of this theory. So far, I could not find any scientific study on this, however, after reviewing average height of people in every country and average consumption of rice in every country, I found an interesting fact – all countries whose people's diet is primarily based on rice, are among shortest nations. Moreover, in those short nations wealthier people are taller on average because they can afford to buy non-rice foods, while poor can only afford to buy the cheapest source of energy food – rice. Well, I hope you got my point.

Proteins

Proteins are the foundation of all life. About one-half of your *dry* body made of protein (about 80% of our *full* body is water). They manage very important activities of the body such as carrying oxygen in the blood and maintaining growth of cells and tissues. Proteins are the building materials for the growth, maintenance, and repair of tissues and muscles. Proteins help your body make hormones including growth hormone.

There are two main sources of protein: *animal* and *vegetable*.

Foods rich in animal protein include beef, fish, chicken, egg whites, and dairy products. Animal products are the richest source of protein, however, eating too much of animal products is attributed to high risks of diseases, including high blood pressure and heart diseases. It mostly caused by raised cholesterol level since animal products are often high in cholesterol and saturated fat. At the same time, animal protein is important as it has a balanced combination of all the amino acids, therefore it is called complete protein. It means you should get your protein from both animal and vegetable products.

There are many vegetables that contain protein, but the richest sources are soy (soybeans, soy milk, soy flour), broccoli, nuts, potatoes, pasta, lentils, oatmeal, rice, chickpeas (garbanzo beans), and navy beans. The most complete source of vegetable protein is soybeans, which I recommend the most.

Proteins should account for 25% to 30% of your diet.

Protein shakes are a good way to reach your daily amount of protein. Follow this recipe:

> *Mix 2 – 5 boiled egg whites (pure protein), 1 to 2 bananas, 3 – 6 strawberries, 1 teaspoon of vanilla in blender at high speed. You can add soy protein or milk or even vegetables. Try different proportions to match your taste. Drink this shake once or twice a day between meals or after exercise, and a smaller shake right before you go to bed.*

Another good recipe:

> *Mix egg whites from hard-boiled eggs and mayonnaise with a little bit of sea salt. Good to eat 3 – 4 times a week.*

Fats

Fats are very important components of our body. They are the *main element in which energy is stored*. Providing insulation from hot and cold, they serve as "shock absorbers" for our organs. To keep your body's chemistry in balance, you should not eliminate all fats. Rather, you want to *eliminate the fats that are bad for your body and include fats that your body needs.*

Fats to avoid are *saturated fats,* which are the type of fat that raises your cholesterol and increases your risk of heart disease. Main sources of saturated fat are the butter fat in milk products and tropical oils such as coconut oil and palm oil. It is fine to have full-fat milk and yogurt, although you might want to go lightly on full-fat cheese. The processing of cheese does make it more fattening to your system than yogurt. In general, *you can easily recognize saturated fats because they will be solid at room temperature.* Saturated fat is also present in red meat; so try to eat less of it, as there are many other great sources of protein that is necessary for us (see chapter "Proteins").

In addition to saturated fat, the hydrogenation process creates another kind of unhealthy fat: *trans fatty acids*, which are made when unsaturated vegetable oils are hydrogenated. To lower your trans fatty acid intake, you should avoid foods that contain ingredients such as margarine, shortening, and hydrogenated or partially hydrogenated oils. Also, you can avoid foods such as french fries, doughnuts, cookies, and crackers, which are often high in trans fatty acids as well as saturated fat (*if you follow my suggestions from "Carbohydrates" chapter above, you will avoid these foods anyway*). Since trans fatty acids rarely occur naturally, they are mostly found in processed foods made with hydrogenated vegetable oil.

Fats that are good for you are **unsaturated fats**. They exist mainly in fish, nuts, seeds and oils from plants. Some examples of foods that contain these fats include tuna, salmon, trout, sardines, herring, avocados, tofu and other soybean products, olives, walnuts, almonds, cashews, pecans, peanuts, sesame seeds and liquid vegetable oils such as olive, soybean, corn, safflower, canola, and sunflower.

Good fats are necessary for our bodies, at the same time we should not consume too much of them. *Total amount of calories that comes from fat should be between 25% and 35% of you daily calories intake.* I understand, it is almost impossible to calculate and fully control this, and you don't need too if you will follow all growth hormone enhancing techniques in this book, because *growth hormone actually reduces extra fat that is stored in your body.*

Everything in our body is connected, and if we try hard enough, even if we do not do everything perfect, most imperfections will be balanced-out, and everything will function normally giving you all possible chances to increase your height.

Potassium

Do you remember the earlier discussion about the importance of salt (sodium) in keeping the water inside each cell of our body? Well, sodium is not the only ingredient that plays such an important function. There is a nutrient that comes from food that we eat, called "potassium" which is stored primarily inside of body cells, and works together with sodium to maintain the extremely important water balance and completeness of each cell in the body.

Sodium does its work primary outside the cell, potassium – inside the cell. Together, they are regulating the movements of water in and out of the cell, and *the right sodium/potassium ratio is crucial to create the right water balance*. This is very important for our health and for our growth.

Moreover, the role of potassium does not stop there. Potassium is essential to many biological reactions including carrying all nutrients into cells and out, controlling the activity of the heart, muscles, nervous system, and just about every living cell in our body, assisting in metabolic processes, transmission of nerve impulses, maintaining the acid-base balance of body's tissues. Potassium activates enzymes for the use of amino acids, it is involved in bone calcification, in the transport of important nutrients into the brain, it is required for protein synthesis. Potassium is also needed to convert the blood sugar into glycogen, which is the body's source of energy (see paragraph "Carbohydrates"). What's even more exiting to know is that *sodium/ potassium ratio directly affects the release of growth hormone*. As you can see, *potassium is essential for life, growth, development, and life span*.

Did I overwhelm you with information that you may not need? I understand, just want you to see the true importance of potassium and make you start thinking about supplying your body with enough potassium.

As you understand the importance of it, also understand that very low level of potassium in the body (potassium deficiency) will not only affect your growth, but also will badly affect health and development of every organ of your body.

Too much of potassium (over 8 gram daily) is also bad and can be toxic and dangerous. That is why I would recommend to be careful with taking supplements that have excessive amount of potassium and consult a doctor if you decide to take such supplements.

Please note, that it is the job of healthy kidneys to keep the right amount of potassium in the body, and when kidneys are not healthy, it is better to limit certain foods, especially supplements that can increase the potassium in the blood to a dangerous level.

If you will just eat more foods that have high content of potassium, it is usually not easy to increase level of potassium to a dangerous level. On average, most people consume too much of sodium but not enough of potassium, especially those that eat a lot of processed foods that almost always have lots of sodium and very little of potassium. In fact, more potassium consumed will help to reduce the amount of sodium in the body.

The **recommended daily potassium intake should be between 3.5 and 5 grams per day.** Since it is almost impossible to get excessive amounts of potassium with regular food, we will avoid calculating. Let's just learn what food we should eat to get enough potassium.

Foods we should eat to get enough potassium

High Potassium Foods	Moderate Potassium Foods
All meats, poultry and fish	Apple juice,
Almonds	Apple sauce
Acorn Squash	Apples
Apricots	Apricots, canned in juice
Avocado	Asparagus
Bananas	Beets
Beans, Baked	Blackberries
Beans, Black	Blueberries
Beans, Refried	Bread and bread products
Broccoli	Broccoli
Brussels sprouts	Butter
Cabbage	Carrots
Cantaloupes	Cauliflower
Carrots	Celery
Chocolate	Cherries
Dates	Coffee
Figs dried	Corn
Granola	Cranberries
Kale	Cucumber
Kiwi	Eggplant
Legumes	Grape Juice
Lentils	Grapefruit
Mango	Grapes
Milk and milk products	Lettuce
Orange juice	Mushrooms
Oranges	Noodles
Winter squash	Okra
Papaya	Onions
Peanut Butter	Parsley
Peanuts	Pasta
Pomegranate	Peach
Pomegranate Juice	Pears
Potatoes	Peas, green
Prune Juice	Peppers
Prunes	Pineapple
Pumpkin	Radish
Pumpkin Seeds	Raspberries
Seeds	Rice
Spinach	Strawberries
Sunflower Seeds	Tangerines
Tomatoes and tomato products	Tea, green
Raisins	Watermelon
Unprocessed natural salt	Wheat bran
Vegetable Juices	Zucchini Squash

As you can see, potassium is readily found in many foods, and the richest sources are unprocessed foods, especially fruits, vegetables, and fresh meats.

If you compare this list to glycemic index (in chapter "Carbohydrates"), you will notice that most foods, with some exceptions, that are high in potassium are low in carbohydrates. It means that *if you will follow the guidelines from chapters "Carbohydrates", "Water", and "Salt", you will create the perfect sodium/potassium/water balance* in your body. *This balance is one of **main secret formulas** to make your body grow and develop with full force.* This should be another reason for you to read again, learn more closely and follow those chapters. It also shows us that *eating wide variety of fresh foods is essential to our development and health.*

It will be worth mentioning that there is another extremely important element called "magnesium" (see next chapter), one of main functions of which is to help holding the potassium inside cells. It means that *even if we consume a lot of potassium, without enough magnesium potassium will not stay inside the cell.* Do you see my dear friend how **everything in our body is connected**? Yes, as important as potassium is for our bodies, it will simply be flashed away without a chance of providing its benefits if there is not enough of magnesium.

Magnesium

As mentioned above, magnesium is a very important essential mineral even though there are only several ounces of it in the body (0.05 percent of body weight). Like potassium, most of magnesium is inside body cells, and concentrated mainly in bones, in the blood, in the liver and kidney, inside the brain and the heart. *This mineral is essential for the metabolism of potassium and sodium*, creating the right balance by removing excess of sodium from the cell and, as mentioned earlier, keeping the potassium in.

Let me stress out how important this is: if there is too little potassium and too much sodium, it creates a big problem – loss of calcium from bones. We will discuss calcium in the next chapter, but I will just say that it is the major part of the bone structure. This means that **magnesium plays a very important role in bone formation and maintenance,** as it forms part of the bone's mineral structure. Simply put, **it is involved in making our bones stronger.**

This shows once again how everything is connected. *All these nutrients are like pieces of the puzzle, working together in harmony as the whole, where magnesium makes this puzzle solvable.*

On top of all that, magnesium is involved in over **300** very important processes inside the body, many of which contribute to production of energy and cardiovascular (blood distribution) function! It also helps regulate blood sugar levels (help prevent diabetes), promotes normal blood pressure, supports a healthy immune system, involved in cell reproduction, and is *necessary for hormonal activity (including growth hormone).* Magnesium is also important in breaking down fats we eat into fatty acids that can be useful in building body parts like nerve passages and cellular membranes.

Just to let you know, if a person at young age constantly has low levels of magnesium, sooner or later in life it may create health problems such as high blood pressure, kidney stones, heart disease, and heart attacks. I don't want to scare you, but I promise – you will not regret if you will take my advices seriously.

All this may probably seem somewhat complicated to you (believe me, there is much more to it, and I'm just trying to cover basics), but my whole idea behind explaining you all this is to show you the importance of magnesium and other nutrients for your health and development. I want you to take it seriously and follow my suggestions if you really want to affect your body's growth.

It is great to know what to do, but it is much better to know why doing it because when you truly believe that what you do will work, it will work always. When somebody tells you what you need to do without explaining why, would you want to do it? Great, so if you didn't understand the importance of magnesium and other nutrients and minerals, read it over because it is crucial.

Let's look into how to make sure we are getting enough magnesium in our diet. First of all, let me point out that on average, in the course of last several decades, most people (especially in the US) do not get enough magnesium, so the chance is – your body may likely need more magnesium to function at its full potential as well.

Usually, about 40-50 percent of the magnesium we consume is absorbed, though this may vary from 25 to 75 percent depending on number of factors. It means that even if you consume a lot of magnesium, a large portion of it will not be absorbed and simply be flashed-out without getting into body's cells. _This is the main reason behind magnesium deficiency, not insufficient intake._

Main factors that _negatively_ affect the absorption of magnesium are: Stress, alcohol, caffeine, smoking, and sugar (another good reason to seriously conceder following suggestions from chapter "Carbohydrates"). Many prescription drugs also known to lower the absorption of magnesium, as well as excessive intake of calcium and fat.

Let me rephrase all this, as it is very important. **Any of the following factors may disturb the balance of magnesium in your body, which can affect your body's development and growth:**

◆ If you worry too much

◆ If you are drinking alcohol

◆ If you consume a lot of caffeine containing products such as coffee, black tee, cola beverages

◆ If you smoke. Smoking causes stress that in turn causes blood cholesterol levels to rise and magnesium levels to fall, making you a special candidate for magnesium deficiency

◆ Eating too much of high-carbohydrate food

◆ Excessive consumption of foods high in fat

Sources of magnesium in food

Almost all of our magnesium sources come from the vegetable kingdom, especially from green vegetables, though seafood has fairly high amounts. Other good sources are: some legumes (beans and peas), nuts, seeds, soy products (especially soy flour and tofu), fruits (especially avocado and dried apricot), brown rice, and whole unrefined grains.

Much of magnesium can be lost in the processing and refining of foods, and in making oils from the magnesium-rich nuts and seeds. Nearly 85 percent of the magnesium in grains is removed when flour is processed. Bread made from whole grain wheat flour provides more magnesium than bread made from white refined flour. Soaking and boiling foods can leach magnesium into the water, so the liquid left from cooking vegetables may be high in magnesium and other minerals.

Another affecting factor is the amount of magnesium in the soil in which the food is grown. Tap water or spring water can be a good source of magnesium along with many other minerals, depending on where the water came from (don't forget the method to clean the water that we have discussed in chapter "Water").

Some food sources of magnesium:

Source	mg/100g*	Source	mg/100g*
Kelp	760	Sunflower seeds	38
Wheat bran	490	Barley	37
Wheat germ	336	Dandelion leaves	36
Almonds	270	Garlic	36
Cashews	267	Fresh green peas	35
Molasses	258	Sweet potato	31
Buckwheat	229	Blackberries	30
Brazil Nuts	225	Broccoli	28
Hazelnuts	184	Cheddar cheese	25
Roasted peanuts	180	Cauliflower	24
Millet	162	Carrots	23
Pecans	142	White fish	23
Rye	115	Celery	22
Bean Curd	111	Chicken	21
Dried Coconut	90	Asparagus	20
Brown rice	88	Beef	18
Whole-wheat bread	76	Potatoes	17
Dried Apricots	62	Tomatoes	14
Corn	48	Oranges	13
Avocado	45	Whole milk	13
Parsley	41	Eggs	12

*mg/100g – Milligrams per 100 grams
For the reference, 110 grams = 4 oz = 1/2 cup = 1/4 lb

For a complete list of foods containing magnesium go to:
www.grow-taller.com/magnesium

As with anything that can benefit you, too much of it can actually be harmful. It applies to magnesium as well. Please look at the table below for **recommended daily amount of magnesium:**

For male <u>under</u> 18 years of age and female <u>under</u> 15 years of age	Weight in pounds X 3	Weight in kilograms X 6.5
For male <u>over</u> 18 years of age and female <u>over</u> 15 years of age	Weight in pounds X 2.5	Weight in kilograms X 5.5

As an example, a 12 years old boy weighting 100 lb (46 kg) should consume about 100 lb X 3 (46 kg X 6.5) = **300 mg** of magnesium per day. This boy may eat slightly over 100 grams of almonds (270 mg per 100 g) for a recommended daily dose of magnesium.

As you can see from both tables above, you should be careful with eating too much of food with high concentration of magnesium, such as nuts. *The best way to meet your daily need for magnesium is to eat a **wide variety** of legumes, nuts, whole grains, and vegetables, not concentrating on a very limited selection.*

Another point I should make is that magnesium (and calcium) is absorbed better when taken between meals (not during or after), before bedtime or on an empty stomach, especially with some vitamin C as ascorbic acid (magnesium requires an acidic stomach environment for best absorption). Therefore, it will be a good idea to grab handful of *different* nuts between meals and before bedtime.

Interestingly enough, all foods recommended for sufficient magnesium consumption are also highly recommended in guidelines from chapter "Carbohydrates". You see, just like with potassium, we are coming back to similar rules to follow, thus it is not as complicated as it seems.

As I mentioned earlier, there is one very important mineral that depends on magnesium and works closely together with it – calcium. **The right calcium-magnesium ratio should be about 10:4 calcium to magnesium.** A good example of this teamwork is that magnesium and calcium work together to make your heart muscle contract in a regular rhythm. If there is a calcium/magnesium imbalance (less magnesium and more calcium), calcium deposits may form on the heart muscle preventing the heart to contract properly.

Magnesium and calcium actually compete with each other. If you take high amounts of calcium daily, you may have a magnesium deficiency, on the contrary – too much magnesium may decrease necessary calcium concentrations. *If you decided take supplements, magnesium and calcium should be taken at different times to allow for better absorption of each of these minerals.*

Calcium

Our bones are made, first of all, from protein in the form of collagen, which is surrounded mainly by calcium and phosphorus (later on that). Together, they make the bone slightly flexible and very strong.

If you want to maintain the height you will gain in this program, for years and years to come, not only you need your bones to grow – you want them to be strong and healthy. Calcium is what will make this possible, as it is one of the most important minerals for the growth, maintenance, and reproduction of the human body. Apart from giving strength to your bones, calcium is necessary for many other functions of the body. Practically every cell in our body, including those in the heart, nerves and muscles, relies on calcium. Calcium is required for muscle contraction and relaxation, which make our movements possible, it maintains normal heartbeat and regulates blood pressure, it is essential for wound healing, and needed for proper functioning of the nervous system.

Calcium is the most abundant mineral in the body. About 99% of it is found in our bones, where it gives them strength. The remaining 1% is found in nerve cells, body tissues, blood, and other body fluids. About 2/3 of bone weight is accounted for by calcium phosphate crystals. Thus, **calcium is regarded as the first nutrient to be provided to ensure optimal bone growth**.

The body does not produce calcium, which means that we must get it from our daily diet. That is why a diet rich in calcium is so important, particularly when bones are growing and developing. Even after full bone development, you still need an adequate calcium intake throughout your life to keep your bones strong and healthy.

In order for your body to function properly, the level of calcium in the blood must stay relatively constant. For this to happen, you need to consume enough calcium throughout the day. Otherwise, your blood will "steal" calcium from your bones to maintain the level it requires. Think of your bones as a "bank". If your diet is low in calcium, your blood "withdraws" the calcium it needs from your bones. When your diet is rich in calcium, you make "deposits" in your calcium "bank". *Over time, if your withdrawals of calcium exceed your deposits, your bones can begin to weaken and become more susceptible to breaking.*

> Keep in mind that smoking, alcohol, and caffeine always have negative impact on bone health, especially if you consume not enough of calcium.

Assuming your calcium intake is sufficient enough, your bones will continue to grow denser until around the age of 30 for men and 25 – 27 for women. After that age, sufficient calcium intake should remains a priority if you want to maintain your bone mass to minimize gradual loss associated with aging. As we get older, we tend to shrink (especially women). This tendency can be prevented through sufficient calcium intake.

In addition, you should know that just like with all other minerals, calcium is not fully absorbed in the body. What is interesting that at younger age the absorption is better than when we get older. In other words, our body takes more calcium from food when we need it the most – when we are young. What's even more interesting, is that the body does this for a reason – *the more calcium we consume and the denser our bones are at the young age, the stronger and healthier our bones will be for the entire length of our life*.

> *The height that you will gain now will not be much affected for your entire life if you will consume enough calcium while you are still young.*

There are several ***other factors that decrease calcium absorption***:

◆ Excessive exercise

◆ Excessive drinking of tea, coffee and soft drinks high in caffeine (cola)

◆ A high protein diet

◆ Liver and kidney disease

◆ Too much salt. As I mentioned earlier, excess sodium and too little potassium causes calcium loss from bones.

◆ Some medications such as diuretics, steroids, anti-seizure medications, immunosuppressive medications, anti-inflammatory drugs (like ibuprofen, naproxen), asthma medication with steroids, and drugs to control heart and blood pressure

◆ Smoking

◆ Alcohol

◆ Low levels of vitamin D (later on that)

Another important point I should emphasize is that to maintain strength, bones need regular physical activity. Exercise helps the body to store calcium in bones, so that the calcium we get from the diet is used more efficiently (another good reason to follow the exercise program I described in detail earlier in the book).

Milk is the food that is most often associated as being high in calcium. It is important to note that there are plenty of other foods that are great sources of calcium though, including other dairy products, many vegetables, calcium enriched orange juice, and other calcium fortified foods. Lets look at them on the following page.

Foods that are good sources of calcium:

Food	One Serving	Calcium
Swiss cheese	2 oz	550 mg
Plain yogurt (low fat)	8 oz	300-450 mg
American cheese	2 oz	350 mg
Goat's milk	1 cup	327 mg
Skim milk	1 cup	315 mg
Buttermilk	1 cup	300 mg
Cow's milk (whole or low fat)	1 cup	300 mg
Soy milk (calcium fortified)	1 cup	300 mg
Rice milk	1 cup	300 mg
Mozzarella cheese	2 oz	300 mg
Orange juice (calcium fortified)	1 cup	300 mg
Cheddar cheese	1.5 oz	300 mg
Plain yogurt (whole milk)	8 oz	275 mg
Black eye peas (boiled)	1 cup	211 mg
Goat cheese	1 oz	200 mg
Figs (dried)	10 fig	169 mg
White beans (dried and cooked)	1 oz	161 mg
Cottage cheese (1% milk fat)	1 cup	138 mg
Spinach (raw)	1 cup	120 mg
Instant oatmeal	1 packet	100 mg
Green peas	1 cup	94 mg
Kale	1 cup of leaves	92 mg
Oranges	1 medium size	72 mg
Almonds (raw)	1 oz (24 nuts)	70 mg
Sweet potatoes (mashed)	1/2 cup	44 mg
Lentils, cooked	1 cup	40 mg
Broccoli (raw)	1 ½ cup	35 mg
Bread, whole wheat or white	1 slice	25 mg
Raisins	1/4 cup	21 mg

*1 oz = 30 g

Any meal that is prepared with above foods will add to your daily calcium requirements.

Keep in mind that the amount of calcium in many prepared foods can vary depending on which brand you buy. Reading food labels and being on the lookout for foods that have at least 20 – 30% daily value of calcium is a good idea. Many other foods, including bread and cereal, may also be fortified with calcium, so check the nutrition facts label to find those brands that are reach in calcium. When looking at food labels, you should know that the percent of calcium daily value shown is based on 1,000 mg, and your suggested daily value of calcium may be different depending on you age (see the table above).

You should know that a large percentage of calcium added to orange juice, rice milk, and soy drinks may settle at the bottom of the carton. This could mean less of the bone-building mineral ends up in your glass until the end of the carton. _Keep the calcium coming steadily by shaking calcium-fortified beverages well before each serving._

Since milk is one of the main sources of calcium and the most popular, lets discuss it in some detail. Let me point-out first of all that cow's milk is not only reach in calcium, but it also contains a large range of naturally occurring nutrients such as vitamin A, vitamin B12, carbohydrate, magnesium, phosphorus, protein, potassium, riboflavin and zinc.

While there are many types of milk available on the market, which milk should we actually drink? Well, simply put, milk that was modified according to some specifications is not as good as plain unprocessed whole milk. The process called "pasteurization" (the milk is heated to high temperature for a period of time) is designed to destroy all disease-carrying germs and increase the shelf life of milk. The problem with this is that most of the good bacteria in pasteurized milk are also destroyed. Moreover, many important nutrients in pasteurized milk are fully or partially destroyed, making their absorption into the body's cells almost impossible. What is most damaging, one of those affected nutrients is calcium, which is damaged and cannot be digested. For that reason, milk producers add vitamin D to the milk to stimulate the calcium absorption.

You should also know that a lot of milk producers feed their cows with unhealthy genetically produced ingredients, including hormones and antibiotics, in order to increase milk production. All these chemicals end-up as part of the milk that we drink, and can bring more harm than benefits. For that reason, I suggest to *drink only milk from cows that were fed only with organically grown feed*. Usually such milk is sold as organic milk. The best milk is from cows that are fed grass, not grain, and allowed to roam free in fields of grass. These cows do not have human pathogens in their milk, but are loaded with beneficial bacteria that assist in the digestion of the milk. The amount of calcium in this type of milk is high and of good quality that the body can actually digest without the aid of vitamin D.

What about low-fat milk? Many people are turning to this type of milk because they want to keep their weight under control. Yes, milk with reduced fat is not reduced in calcium because the calcium is not contained in the fat portion of milk, so removing the fat will not affect the calcium content, as well as most other nutrients. However, as we discussed earlier in the chapter "Fats", fat is an important component of our body, therefore we should not completely avoid it. Also, *the process of reducing fat in milk destroys natural vitamin D contained in it*.

If you will follow the program I laid-out for you in this book, especially exercise, proper water and salt intake, and recommendations on the diet, your body will function properly, and the fat from milk should not make you any fatter. For that reason I suggest to avoid low-fat or no-fat (skim) milk. Keep in mind also that when all the fat is removed from milk – it does not look and does not taste like milk. For that reason, milk producers add white paint and chemical substances to adjust color and taste, so you would think that you drink real milk. Many people develop allergies from such milk mainly because of added ingredients.

Even if you will drink the best possible milk to reach your calcium requirements, I suggest not only relying on milk for calcium, but also on other dairy and non-dairy foods that contain calcium (see table above).

If a person does not receive enough calcium over a long period of time, he can develop calcium deficiency, which leads to osteoporosis, hypertension, and other disorders.

A little bit of caution: keep in mind that even though calcium should be an absolutely necessary part of your diet, too much of it taken over long periods of time may create some unwelcome side effects later in life, such as increased risk of kidney stones in some people. Too much calcium can also block the absorption of iron, zinc and manganese – other very important nutrients, as well as magnesium (we just mentioned earlier). For that reason, let me give you suggested **daily calcium requirements** for all ages:

Age	Calcium intake per day
0 – 6 months	210 mg (less than 1 serving of milk)
7 – 12 months	270 mg (about 1 servings of milk)
1 – 3 years old	500 mg (about 2 servings of milk)
4 – 8 years old	800 – 1200 mg (about 3 – 4 cups of milk)
9 – 18 years old	1300 mg (about 4 cups of milk)
19 – 50 years old	1000 mg (about 3.5 cups of milk)
51 and over	1200 – 1500 mg (about 4 – 5 cups of milk)

*1 cup = 8 ounces

Lets not forget that calcium intake is just one component of the complex dynamics regulating calcium balance, and as important as calcium is, it cannot be utilized without presence of correct amounts of magnesium (see chapter "magnesium") and phosphorus (see chapter "phosphorus"). Also, as previously mentioned, there is another ingredient that directly affects the calcium absorption – vitamin D.

Vitamin D

We have already discussed vitamin D in the chapter "Affects of Sunlight". Yes, the majority of vitamin D we get is produced inside our skin when exposed to direct ultraviolet light of the Sun.

Nothing can substitute the exposure to sunlight as it affects not only the production of vitamin D but also many other crucial processes in our body. Interestingly enough, when you receive your vitamin D from Sun exposure your body can self-regulate and substantially reduce vitamin D production if the body had enough of it. This makes it very difficult to overdose on vitamin D from the exposure to the Sun. Nevertheless, if you do not get enough of vitamin D, your bones become wick and cannot grow at full potential. Keep in mind that synthetic sunscreens that block ultraviolet rays also block vitamin D production inside the skin.

Vitamin D is essential for life, as its major biological function is to regulate the calcium metabolism by stimulating the absorption of calcium from food, participating in getting this absorbed calcium into our bones, and maintaining its normal levels. Vitamin D's other functions include controlling absorption of phosphorus (will be discussed in a later chapter), magnesium and other minerals, regulating critical functions of many types of cells in the body including our brain cells (yes, our brain development is linked to presence of vitamin D), playing a role in controlling blood pressure, and preventing artery damage.

Luck of vitamin D in the body over long period of time may lead not only to weakened bones and stunned growth, but also to several other potential problems later in life, such as a weakened immune system, increased risk of cancer, diabetes, multiple sclerosis, and heart disease. I'm not writing this to scare you, just want you to be aware of this and be outside under the sun more often.

Insufficient amounts of vitamin D is also one of the main reason for the most frequent childhood disease in many developing countries today, called "rickets", which softens bones, potentially leading to fractures and bone deformation. In fact, during the Industrial Revolution, rickets became epidemic in places where the pollution from factories blocked the sun's ultraviolet rays. At that time scientists figured-out the real cause of rickets (vitamin D deficiency), and governments of some countries had pushed milk producers (most common drink) to add vitamin D to their product. That initiative alone completely eliminated the epidemic in those countries, which shows how important and powerful this vitamin is.

Now, since it is not always possible for everybody to get enough of direct sunlight exposure, especially in some parts of the world where sunlight is often limited during some periods of the year, there are other ways to get the vitamin D similar to what the skin produces – supplements and food.

As you probably noticed, nowhere in this book I suggest using supplements. It does not mean that supplements are not good for you; its just not all supplements are created equally, including supplements with vitamin D in them. There are limitless of different manufacturers for these supplements, and all of them have their own way of creating those. How do we know which supplements are better made, better absorbed into the body, and have no side effects? Well, why do we even need to think about it when we have much better, completely safe and natural ways of getting all necessary vitamins and minerals? Therefore, lets discuss _only food sources_ of vitamin D.

Let me just point-out that there are two types of vitamin D exist – vitamin D2 and vitamin D3. Vitamin D2 is synthetically produced by chemical procedures, and vitamin D3 is produced from animal sources (mainly extracted from sheep's wool). Vitamin D3 is very similar to what our skin produces under ultraviolet light of the sun, and is 4 – 5 times more effective than vitamin D2. Both types of vitamin D are used by different manufacturers in different food products. If the vitamin D is added, it is usually shown on the label which type was used. Therefore, avoid food products with added vitamin D2, and get only with vitamin D3.

As you already know, most commercially produced milk is fortified with vitamin D3 (in US and Canada, not in Europe). As I mentioned earlier, lowering fat in milk reduces vitamin D. You should also understand that even when good quality vitamin D artificially added to the low fat milk, this vitamin D does not dissolve in water. It needs fat in order to enter the body. It all means it has to be *whole milk* to be effective. Keep in mind also that most fortified soy beverages contain vitamin D2, not D3.

Dairy products made from milk, such as cheese, yogurt, and ice cream are generally *not* fortified with vitamin D. Only a few foods naturally contain significant amounts of vitamin D, including fatty fish and fish oils. The table below lists most of them.

Good sources of natural vitamin D

Food	Serving Size	IU per serving*
Herring	85 g (3 ounces)	1383
Cod liver oil, pure (not refined)	1 Tablespoon	1,360
Sockeye salmon, cooked	100 g (3.5 oz)	646
Catfish	85 g (3 oz)	425
Salmon, cooked	100 g (3.5 oz)	360
Mackerel, cooked	100 g (3.5 oz)	345
Tuna fish, canned in oil	85 g (3 oz)	200
Sardines, canned in oil, drained	50 g (1.75 oz)	250
Milk, vitamin D fortified	1 cup	98
Margarine, vitamin D fortified	1 Tablespoon	60
Pudding, with vitamin D fortified milk	1/2 cup	50
Ready-to-eat cereals fortified with vitamin D	3/4 – 1 cup	40
Egg (egg yolk)	1 whole	20
Beef liver, cooked	100 g (3.5 oz)	15
Cheese, Swiss	1 ounce	12

* *(IU) International Units*

Current government dietary guideline for humans is to consume 200 IU of vitamin D per day for everyone from infants up to the age of 51, and 400 IU for people over 51. These numbers however are sufficient enough to avoid rickets, but not necessarily enough to support good health and strong bones. *A 20-minute full-body exposure to summer sun will trigger the delivery of up to 20,000 units of vitamin D in people with lighter skin and up to 10,000 units in people with darker skin.* This clearly shows that what government guideline recommends is *not enough*, and that in normal natural environment, before industrial revolution, humans were always getting much more of vitamin D than today.

There are many studies being conducted today that are trying to figure all the benefits of vitamin D, and what daily intake of it should actually be enough. Majority of studies suggest that **daily vitamin D intake should be between 1,000 and 2,000 units**, *plus spending at least 10 to 15 minutes in the sun.*

Just to throw another reason to pay attention to my recommendations on vitamin D, there was a study published in the Archives of Internal Medicine in September 2007 with an analysis of 18 randomized controlled trials involving 57,000 people over the age of 50. That study found that people who took at least 500 IU of vitamin D daily had *7% lower risk of death.* Lead researcher in that study, Dr. Philippe Autier suggested that *vitamin D may block cancer cell development and improve immune system functions.*

As we can see, milk alone is not enough to get your dally dose of vitamin D, so if you want to be healthy and grow taller, expose yourself to the sun more often (read chapter "Affects of Sunlight") and follow food recommendation shown in the table above.

Vitamin C

In addition to other nutrients, vitamin C (ascorbic acid) is also *required for optimal bone metabolism*. It is needed for the synthesis and formation of collagen, which is the main organic component of bone, and for the synthesis of other essential elements of the bone and cartilage. It means that your bones do need sufficient amounts of vitamin C to develop properly.

On top of all that, vitamin C is one of most important vitamins for our general health, as it is essential for the formation, growth, and repair of not only bones, but also skin, and connective tissue which binds other tissues and organs together. Vitamin C helps the body to absorb iron, which is needed to make red blood cells. It helps to maintain healthy teeth and gums, heal wounds and burns, and protects cells against damage by free radicals (bad molecules in the body). It is also involved in the brain function, affects the mood, plays a role in converting fat into energy, involved in the metabolism of cholesterol, and positively affects our immune system.

Unlike with vitamin D, our body does not have the ability to make its own vitamin C, and too little of it can lead to some major problems. Therefore, we must obtain this important vitamin through our diet. The body also cannot store vitamin C, and leftovers of the vitamin leave the body through the urine. That means – you always need to include this vitamin in your diet.

While the recommended by United States Government's National Academy of Sciences daily intake of vitamin C is 75 – 90 mg for adults and 40 – 75 mg for children, higher amounts should not give any negative side effects, and usually *up to 2,000 mg per day is safe*. Therefore, we can see that it is practically impossible to overdose on vitamin C by dietary sources alone.

Sources of Vitamin C:

Virtually all fruits and vegetables contain vitamin C, just in different amounts. Table below shows the most vitamin C rich foods:

Food	Mg of vitamin C per 100 grams of food
Rosehips	1,500 – 2,000
Guava, tropical	183
Blackcurrant	155 – 215
Kiwifruit, yellow	120 – 180
Kiwifruit, green	98
Papaya	62
Redcurrant	58 – 81
Strawberry	57
Orange	53
Lemon juice	46
Melon, cantaloupe	42
Grapefruit	34
Melon, honeydew	25
Mango	28
Raspberry	27
Tomato	19 – 40
Pineapple	15
Grape, european	11
Watermelon	10
Apricot	10
Plum	10
Blueberry	8

As you already know well, all these fruits and vegetables are absolutely necessary for many other reasons, not only because of vitamin C in them. Therefore, if you eat enough fruits and vegetables, and *wide variety* of them every day, you should not worry about getting enough of vitamin C. However, if you don't eat enough of fruits and vegetables, supplementations may be necessary. In such case ask your doctor what is best for you.

Keep in mind that not eating enough fresh fruits and vegetables can cause the deficiency of vitamin C, which not only can affect bone growth, but can make a person feel tired, weak, and irritable, can decrease wound healing, cause nosebleeds, weakened tooth enamel, and decrease resistance to infections. Severe deficiency of vitamin C, called "scurvy", causes bruising, gum and dental problems, dry skin and hair, and anemia. So, let's eat some fruits my friend, and you will be rewarded with good health and increased height.

Vitamin K

Another vitamin that ***plays an important role in bone formation*** is vitamin K. It activates several important proteins that are involved in the health of our bones (triggers the ability of those proteins to bind calcium). Low levels of vitamin K circulating in the body have been linked to low bone density, and increased intake of vitamin K shown improvements in bone health. Even though this vitamin's main function is to play an important role in the process of blood clotting, it does also affect our body's growth, so we should make sure we have it in our body.

Vitamin K is stored in the fat tissue of the human body, in very small amounts, constantly flashing it out. It means that *if you are not constantly supplying your body with vitamin K, your body can quickly loose it completely.*

Vitamin K is found mainly in green, leafy vegetables. The richest sources of this vitamin are: kale, collards, spinach, beet greens, brussels sprouts, turnip greens, and broccoli. See table on the following page.

Most foods containing Vitamin K:

Alfalfa	Collards	Marjoram	Rhubarb
Amaranth leaves	Coriander	Mayonnaise	Sage
Asparagus	Cucumber	Milk	Sauerkrauts
Basil	Dandelion greens	Mustard greens	Sea kelp
Beet greens	Dried Spices	Okra	Soy bean
Bread crumbs	Endive	Olive oil	Soybean oil
Broccoli	Enriched egg	Onions	Spinach
Brussels sprouts	noodles	Oregano	Thyme
Cabbage	Fish oils	Parsley	Turnip greens
Cauliflower	Kale	Peas	Yogurt
Celery flakes	Lettuce	Plums	
Chard	Liver	Prunes	

There are no particular amounts of vitamin K I will recommend. All you need is to include at least small amounts of green, leafy vegetables in your diet *every day*. Your body does not need a lot of vitamin K, but it will suffer without it.

Zinc

Zinc is a metallic element, which is found in almost every cell of human body. It is absolutely vital to living, and even a small deficiency can cause health problems. ***Zinc is one of the major elements involved in human growth process***. It is a mineral that is required for numerous functions in the body, such as carbon dioxide exchange, bio-chemical synthesis of DNA, RNA (another very important molecule) and protein. Zinc is necessary for normal growth of all cells and tissues as it affects individual cell multiplying, and aids in regulating hormones. Zinc protects all the cells in the body and their membranes from bad viruses. Zinc also regulates metabolism of very important minerals – copper, magnesium, manganese, and selenium that more or less directly participate in body growth regulation.

When cells and tissues don't have enough zinc, many problems can arise: delayed healing of wounds, weak development of bones and muscles, as well as the nervous system. Luck of zinc can delay puberty (sexual development), induce very rapid loss of hair and deformation in the nails, allergies, loss of appetite, weight loss, loss of the sense of taste as well as smell, impaired vision, but what is even more dangerous – weaken immune responses.

Everybody should know that **_getting sufficient amounts of zinc is a way to boost the immune system at any age_**. It means that even common cold and many other diseases may be prevented or treated with increased zinc intake. Just keep in mind that zinc is not medication, and zinc level is not the only factor that plays a role in treating or preventing diseases. Zinc deficiency can also be a factor in birth defects and low birth weight, which can also affect the future final height of a child.

Another important fact we need to know is that luck of _zinc can lead to a greatly reduced absorption of nutrients from food_. It means that **_even if you eat enough foods with many other important nutrients, without zinc those nutrients simply will not get into your body in necessary amounts_**.

Our body does not store zinc, as zinc is constantly lost through sweat and food processing, so you should intake sufficient amounts of it every day if you want to be healthy and maximize your height.

Now, lets learn how much zinc you need and where to get it from.

Recommended daily intake of zinc:

Age	mg per day
Birth to 6 months	3
6 to 12 months	5
1 to 11 years	10
11+ years	15

Pregnant and breastfeeding women should have about 7 mg more per day than what is recommended for others.

Just for your information, you may find from other sources that recommended dietary allowance (RDA) for zinc is lower than numbers above. All you need to know is that RDA is the minimum dosage recommended, but not ideal.

Also, it is very important to know that *significant overdose of zinc may be very harmful* and can lead to many serious health problems, one of which is weakened immune system, so those who take supplements should be very careful. *Doses per day should not be larger than 5 mg for children under 1 year old, 15 mg – under 11, and 25 mg for 11 years old and up.*

Great sources of zinc are found in red meat, poultry and seafood. While grains, dairy products, beans, nuts, eggs, cereals, seeds and brewer's yeast also supply good quality zinc, however zinc absorption is more effective if it comes from animal proteins than from plant sources. For this reason, vegetarians need to eat more zinc to ensure that they don't become deficient.

Use the following table and recommended zinc daily intake as your guide.

Zinc content in food:

Food	Serving size	mg per serving
Mollusks, oyster, wild, raw,	6 medium	76
Cereals ready-to-eat, Wheat Bran	3/4 cup	15
Cereals ready-to-eat, Corn Flakes	1-1/3 cup	15
Cereals ready-to-eat, Whole Grain	3/4 cup	15
Cereals ready-to-eat, Raisin Bran Flakes	1 cup	15
Turkey neck, all classes, meat only, cooked	1 neck	11
Beef shanks, cooked	3 ounces	8.7
Crab, Alaska king, cooked	3 ounces	6.5
Chicken giblets, cooked	1 cup	6.1
Beef rib, trimmed to 1/4" fat, cooked, roasted	3 ounces	5.9
Beans, baked, canned, plain or vegetarian	1 cup	5.8

Barley, pearled, raw	1 cup	4.3
Lamb, trimmed to 1/4" fat, cooked	3 ounces	4.2
Turkey, dark meat, cooked, roasted	3 ounces	3.8
Buckwheat flour, whole-groat	1 cup	3.7
Chicken leg, roasted,	1 leg	2.7
Lobster, cooked	3 ounces	2.5
Baked beans, canned	½ cup	1.7
Cashews, dry roasted	1 ounce	1.6
Yogurt, fruit, low fat	1 cup	1.6
Chickpeas	½ cup	1.3
Fish, tuna salad	1 cup	1.2
Oat bran, cooked	1 cup	1.1
Cheese, Swiss	1 ounce	1.1
Almonds, dry roasted	1 ounce	1.0
Milk, whole	1 cup	0.9
Chicken breast, roasted, with skin removed	1/2 breast	0.9
Cheese, cheddar or mozzarella,	1 ounce	0.9
Fish, salmon, sockeye, cooked	1/2 fillet	0.8
Peas, boiled,	1/2 cup	0.8
Rice, white, cooked	1 cup	0.7

For a complete list of foods containing zinc go to:
www.grow-taller.com/zinc

Keep in mind: some foods shown on that list are not necessarily good for you. If you've read everything in this book up until this point, I'm sure you know already what is good for you, and what is not. As we discussed previously, ***there are no strict rules on your diet, just guidelines***, *and you have a lot of choices within those guidelines.*

As you can see from the table above, the best natural source of zinc is oysters, and they have much more zinc that you need in just few pieces. It does not mean you should avoid them, just eat them not too often. It is Ok to overdose on zinc once in a while, what counts is the average amount of it you consume over time.

As you are trying to calculate your zinc intake, you should also keep in mind that zinc that gets inside the body is not necessarily absorbed fully. There are several factors that affect the absorption of zinc. The absorption can be decreased by high fiber diets, as well as by the presence of phytates (phosphorus compounds that are found in legumes, cereals, and grain breads). This is the reason why zinc from animal foods (typically low in fiber and phytates) have four times greater bio-availability compared to plant foods. This factor is not a reason to eat less fiber, even if the fiber can decrease zinc absorption. As we will discuss in the following chapter, plant based fiber is necessary for human health and growth and is comparable to zinc in its usefulness.

Whole grains are a better source of zinc than refined grains as they have the ability to produce enzymes that can destroy phytates.

Other factors affecting zinc level:

♦ Zinc absorption in the body is decreased by the constant consumption of high protein diets, lemon juice, and especially large amounts of alcohol.

♦ Zinc is lost in cooking some foods even under the best conditions. To retain zinc, cook foods in a minimal amount of water and for the shortest possible time.

♦ Zinc is lost through excessive sweating.

♦ Zinc absorption can be increased by increasing intake of vitamins C, E and B6 and minerals such as magnesium

♦ Use of several types of medications.

Now, you would ask me, how can I consume exactly the amount that I need? Well, just as with other vitamins and nutrients we have already discussed, there are two ways to control the right balance – by eating recommended food containing zinc or taking supplements. As you well know already, I prefer to stay out from any supplements if possible, because the right food is the best possible source of all vitamins and minerals.

Yes, it is much more difficult to figure how much of this mineral you have consumed with diet alone, especially when you have to take into account all other vitamins and nutrients, but don't worry, you don't have to do exact amounts. All you need is just to be aware of what your body needs and to try to be as close as you can to these recommendations, but don't "go crazy" on that. *Your body has the ability to regulate the absorption of zinc according to its needs.* As the matter of fact, **a well-balanced diet with which you take different variety of foods recommended throughout this program, is good enough to get enough zinc, achieve great results in gaining height, to become strong and healthy for the rest of your life.**

Parents of a newborn should know that breast milk is the optimal source of nutrition during infancy, and one of the most important benefits of breastfeeding is that it is the best possible source of zinc for infants. This is because zinc is available in highest quantities in breast milk and absorbed most easily. More on that in chapter "Suggestions for parents of newborn".

The following information is extremely important, especially for parents whose children have GH deficiency: according to several studies, *about half of all children with Growth Hormone deficiency have also zinc deficiency.* When these children are treated with daily zinc supplementation during several months, their body's growth rate significantly increases. What was also found is that children with GH deficiency and normal zinc level did not benefit from increased zinc supplementation. This means that *if a child had been diagnosed with GH deficiency, I strongly suggest checking child's zinc level in the blood*, and if zinc deficiency is found, definitely discuss what you learned here with a doctor and make sure a child receives enough zinc from now on. I suggest doing that even without knowing if a child has GH deficiency, but grow at very slow pace.

There is a relatively simple and accurate way to check if a person has zinc deficiency. It is done by simply tasting the 0.1 % water solution of zinc. Just mix 1 gram of zinc sulfate in 1 litter (0.26 gallons) of distilled water, take a sip of the solution (approximately 5 – 10 ml) and rinse it in the mouth for exactly ten seconds, spiting it out after that. You can tell if you have enough zinc in your body by feeling the flavor of the solution. You must not eat or drink for at least one hour before the test, and the solution must be room temperature.

This zinc taste test can have four different results:

1. No specific taste sensation: tastes like plain water. This indicates a major deficiency

2. No immediate taste is noticed, but within the ten seconds of the test, a 'dry' or 'metallic' or 'sweet' taste is experienced. This indicates a moderate deficiency

3. An immediate slight taste is noted, which increases within few seconds. This indicates a deficiency of minor degree

4. An immediate, strong and unpleasant taste is experienced. This indicates a good sign that that no zinc deficiency exists.

This test is non-toxic and can be performed with children of any age. I suggest doing it especially by those children that are much shorter than their peers. It will not hurt for an adult to do this test as well.

Another way to find-out zinc level is by using "Zinc Talley" – a nutritional test that can be found in health food stores.

Fiber

Fiber is made up of many compounds, mostly special type of carbohydrates that cannot be digested or broken down into nutrients in the stomach, found mainly in the outer layers of plants.

Fiber is very important for health because it has great positive influence on our digestion process. The health benefits of a diet rich in fiber include lower cholesterol and a reduced risk of heart disease and certain cancers. What's important for us is that *fiber plays an important role in body's growth and development by affecting the release of growth hormone*.

In the chapter "Dieting Strategies" for growth hormone increase we discussed about insulin that produced in the body with the help of carbohydrates. Insulin is an important hormone that encourages your body to burn carbohydrates for energy, but what it also does is decreasing the release of growth hormone into the body. That is where fiber plays an important role – by keeping insulin levels down, which in turn keeps growth hormone levels up. Fiber is what we need – another tool at our disposal to increase growth hormone level.

Fiber can be found in a variety of foods, including wheat, potatoes, nuts, and certain fruits and vegetables. Recommended amount of fiber is 20 to 35 grams a day for adults. For children up to age of 18, the recommended daily dose (in grams) is determined by adding five to a child's age. For example, a 14-year-old would need $14 + 5 = 19$ grams of fiber per day.

Food sources high in fiber:

	Serving size	Fiber (g)
Fruits		
Raspberries	1 cup	8
Pear, with skin	1 medium	5.5
Apple, with skin	1 medium	4.4
Strawberries (halves)	1 1/4 cup	4
Banana	1 medium	3
Orange	1 medium	3
Apricots dried	2 halves	1.7
Figs, dried	2 medium	1.6
Raisins	2 tablespoons	1
Legumes, nuts & seeds		
Split peas, cooked	1 cup	16
Baked beans, cooked	1 cup	16
Black beans, cooked	1 cup	15
Lentils, cooked	1 cup	15
Lima beans, cooked	1 cup	13
Sunflower seed kernels	1/4 cup	4
Almonds	1 ounce	3.5
Pistachio nuts	1 ounce	3
Pecans	1 ounce	2.7
Vegetables		
Artichoke, cooked	1 medium	10
Peas, cooked	1 cup	9
Broccoli, boiled	1 cup	5
Turnip greens, boiled	1 cup	5
Sweet corn, cooked	1 cup	5
Brussels sprouts, cooked	1 cup	4
Potato, with skin, baked	1 medium	4
Tomato paste	1/4 cup	2.7
Carrot, raw	1 medium	1.7
Grains, cereal & pasta		
Spaghetti, whole-wheat	1 cup	6
Barley, pearled, cooked	1 cup	6
Bran flakes	3/4 cup	5
Oat bran muffin	1 medium	5
Oatmeal, cooked	1 cup	4
Popcorn, air-popped	3 cups	3.5
Brown rice, cooked	1 cup	3.5
Bread, rye	1 slice	2
Bread, whole-wheat	1 slice	2

For a complete list of foods containing fiber go to:
www.grow-taller.com/fiber

Keep in mind that fiber doesn't work properly without water. The more fiber you consume, the more water your body needs to normally process all the food that you eat. This is another good reason to follow my suggestions on water intake in the chapter "Water". Also, raw or slightly cooked vegetables will provide an excellent source of fiber. However, overcooking vegetables may reduce their fiber content.

As with everything else, overdose on fiber (taken in excess of 60 to 70 grams daily) has the potential to cause harm.

My dear friend, don't be frustrated if you feel you are getting too much information. Many of these high fiber foods are also low in carbohydrates, which is, as we have learned already, great for your body's development. It means that ***you have great selection of foods to choose from to get all the necessary ingredients to succeed in your quest to grow taller.*** My most important goal is to bring the importance of all this to your attention. As you can see, ***there are no strict rules; all you have to do is to try to stay within recommended guidelines***, and you will be just fine. Simply put, *eating balanced meals containing whole grain, fresh fruits and vegetables will ensure enough fiber in your diet.*

Phosphorus

We have discussed phosphorus earlier in the section "Calcium". Phosphorus together with calcium surrounds collagen proteins in our bones, forming bones' structure, making them strong, and at the same time slightly flexible to prevent fractures. We also learned that *without the presence of enough phosphorus, calcium couldn't be utilized well.* In other words, calcium alone cannot build strong bones and tissues. It needs phosphorus to maximize its bone-strengthening benefits. You see, ***every process in our body is like teamwork of many small ingredients where each one plays its own role, and phosphorus is an important part of that team***.

What is phosphorus? It is a mineral that is abundant in human body (about 400-700 grams of it), and only second in mass after calcium. Nearly 3/4 of phosphorus is combined with the calcium in bones and teeth, in a compound known as calcium phosphate – the source of bone strength. The remaining phosphorus is combined mainly with nitrogen to metabolize fats and carbohydrates in other tissues.

Phosphorus is the main element in the structure of all tissue cells, and an important component in nerve and muscle tissues (keeps muscles and nerves working properly). It is vitally important for the normal metabolism of numerous compounds in the body. Phosphorus helps our kidneys effectively excreting wastes, helps maintain good teeth, gives our body a lot of energy, keeps the mind alert and active, it forms the proteins that aid in reproduction, and may even help block cancer. What is even more interesting, phosphorus also helps stimulate our glands to release hormones.

Why do you need to know all that? What's in it for you? Well, you don't need to remember everything here, we are not studying biology, but you do need to understand the importance of phosphorus, at least because *it plays a big role in our bones' health*. And healthy bones do grow better.

Even though phosphorus deficiency is rare, you should know that not getting enough phosphorus can contribute to many health problems, such as bone problems, stress and anxiety, general weakness, fatigue, irregular breathing, numbness, skin sensitivity, teeth weakness, loss of weight, and many other problems. Phosphorus deficiency results in bone loss just as calcium deficiency does.

As you already know well, too much of any nutrient can be very toxic. This rule applies to phosphorus as well. It is possible to overdose on phosphorus, especially if you are taking supplements. Also, most soft drinks are loaded with phosphorous, so *it could be a real problem if you drink a lot of soda*. Too much phosphorus is also contained in most *junk foods*. Phosphorus toxicity can result in diarrhea, nausea, vomiting, and other problems. However *the biggest problem excess of phosphorous can bring is that it can block calcium formation in bones.*

At the same time, taking large amounts of calcium can interfere with phosphorus absorption. You see, *phosphorus and calcium work together as partners to form strong and healthy bones*, but too much of either nutrient can disturb the balance in that partnership that will affect bones growth. What does it all tell you? Well, eat healthy according to recommendations in this book, and please, *avoid junk foods and sodas.*

Thankfully, getting enough phosphorus in our body is not a big issue because there is plenty of it in foods, and it's unlikely that you are not getting enough of it. It is especially abundant in *milk, meat, fish, grains cereals and green vegetables*. Other vegetables such as carrots, and fruits such as black currants, raspberries, raisins, and apricots are also fairly good sources. Other sources of this mineral are soybeans, lentils, and other pulses and legumes.

If you will follow suggestions on food intake from previous chapters, you will be just fine on getting enough of phosphorus. Therefore, we will not get into more detailed description of recommended foods containing phosphorus.

Recommended intakes of phosphorous are about the same as for calcium so that a one-to-one ratio is maintained:

- Infants: 240-360 mg
- Children: 800-1200 mg
- Adults: 800 mg

Both calcium and phosphorus are found naturally in dairy products, but most calcium supplements and calcium-fortified foods and beverages don't contain phosphorus. Also, phosphorus from animal sources is absorbed greater than from cereals and legumes. It does not mean you should eat more meat because of that. In fact, since meat is so rich in phosphorous, eating too much meat can also block calcium formation.

As we can see, *it is all about balance*, which is not a perfect science, and all we have to do is to search for that balance to the best of our abilities. How will you know when you have that balance? Simple. *If you feel healthy, strong and energized for a long time, if you rarely get sick, and gain height more rapidly (when you are still young enough), most likely you do have that balance.* And when you have it, try to maintain it at all times.

Other nutrients

There are many other vitamins and minerals that we did not discuss in this book simply because they are not relevant enough for our main subject. However, it does not mean that those nutrients are irrelevant to our health. Just to name a few important ones such as vitamin E, vitamin B and its variety, vitamin A, Fluoride, Selenium, Iron and Copper, each playing an important role in our body's development and general health. Yes, even if the nutrient is not directly involved in the process of human growth, it is involved indirectly. If you've read everything up until this point, you already know how everything in our body is connected, how every organ and every process depend on other organs and processes. It means that **everything you do to make yourself healthier, including consuming foods with all vitamins and minerals will also maximize your body's growth.**

Other important suggestions about food

We need all vitamins and minerals, but how do we get them all? The answer is easy: follow suggestions for food intake in this book, and always try to have **maximum variety of foods** I recommend. If you do that, your body will be supplied with all necessary ingredients. *If you eat very limited variety of foods, even if these foods are highly recommended in this book, it is almost definite that you will lack some necessary nutrients and vitamins for you body's growth and development.*

What about proportions? – You would ask. How do we know exactly how much of each vitamin and mineral our body needs and how to control it? First of all, read all the suggestions above. However, you cannot know exactly how much of each ingredient your body needs, not to mention – precisely how much of each food to consume. There are so many factors involved in the process, such as: different absorption of different ingredients, quality of food, what time of the day and of the year you take that food, your physical condition, your mood while you eat, and many other factors that make it seemingly impossible to do exactly what your body needs and can be quite confusing.

Thankfully, our body is an incredible mechanism, which helps us resolve this seemingly impossible task. To work properly, all it needs is you trying your best to supply it with all necessary ingredients in amounts that are approximate to what is good for the body. Our brain then will figure out the rest. It will regulate how much of each ingredient will be absorbed, working like the most powerful computer ever existed. This is especially true for someone who eats a well-rounded diet based on *natural* whole foods such as fruits, vegetables, meat and fish, but not for people who use a lot of supplements which can be very misleading.

Let me point out one important factor that significantly affects how your body absorbs food and how well your body will react to the much-improved quality of your diet. Do you remember what we have discussed in the chapter "Water"? Remember, how water that we drink reacts to our thoughts and feelings? Yes, that rule applies to food as well. If you missed or did not fully understand how it happens, I strongly suggest reading chapters "The power of thought" and "Water" again. All the benefits from the food that we consume depend very much on what we actually think of that food.

As strange as it may sound to some people, *food as any other substance has its own energy, not only from its chemical composition but from the universe of virtual energy that surrounded that food from the moment of its creation till you eat it, and even after.* That virtual energy can be transformed from one object to another, from one living organism to another. It means that *virtual energy of food depends on the energy of the place where it was made or grown, and the energy of those who made that food,* and in case of meat – how animals were slaughtered. This is another good reason to buy natural whole foods, especially directly from farmers.

Why do you think most vegetarians don't eat meat or fish? Not only because they are against killing animals. Many vegetarians understand that negative energy from animal's pain and agony in the moment of slaughtering where left in its meat, and when eaten, that energy can be transferred to the person who ate it. It is actually true, and many farmers who understand this issue are trying to do it as humanly as possible, making sure that the slaughtering process goes completely painless and fearless for animals. In Jewish culture for example, this is how animals were slaughtered for thousands of years.

You should know that what can be even more damaging to a person is feeling of guilt for eating animal food, because energy of that thought alone is very negative and powerful. Therefore, *when you eat meat or any other food, think of that food as something good and necessary for you, think of it as it is full of good energy that will fill-up your entire body making you joyful and healthy.* This way, even if the food is not from the best source and not of the best quality, it will be much more beneficial than food that you are feeling guilty eating, even of good quality and from the healthiest source.

If you are not enjoying certain foods, even if you know it is good for your health, I usually suggest to skip it, *don't force yourself.* There are some exceptions of course, but for most of us there are plenty of choices to get all necessary ingredients for your body from many different sources we have discussed in this book. I will repeat myself by saying that there are no strict rules in this program, only guidelines. And one of most important guidelines – **try to fully enjoy your meals, think of every bite that you eat and every sip of water that you drink as something magical that makes your body even healthier and growing at full force**.

Remember, our diet in childhood has a major effect on how strong we are as adults. What you eat during your whole life will affect how able you will be to repair bones that you are trying so hard to grow today, as well as cartilage, ligaments, tendons, and muscles in events of damage and natural wear and tear.

Besides proper food intake, our organism needs something else to be able to function at its best: it needs to be in good physical and mental shape. After reading this book, I'm sure you know exactly what it means and how to accomplish that – **follow mental and physical exercises described here and you will have all pieces of a puzzle laid-out perfectly to maximize your growth and live long, happy and healthy life**.

Suggestions for parents of newborn

If you are a young person, reading this book only for your own benefits, you can skip this chapter, but if you are a parent of a newborn or planning to be, and care how your child's body will grow and develop, read on.

Parents of a newborn should know that child's health during his or her entire life, as well as child's future final height very much depends on nutrition a child gets before he or she is born, and first days and years of his or her life. Therefore, **it is parents' responsibility for their child's future health, height, even longevity of child's life**, and providing all the necessary nutrients to a child should be a priority.

Information for expected mothers

Starting from conception, expected mother should have a diet that contains everything that a child needs. *If the mother is lacking in any vitamins and nutrients, her baby might lack them too.* I strongly suggest expected mother to read food suggestions in this book, at the same time checking with her doctor for additional suggestions, and if she is lacking on any necessary vitamins and minerals. One of the main rules to follow is to include as *larger variety* of foods as possible to ensure that every necessary vitamin and mineral is available in the body for both mother and the baby. In other words, an every day well-balanced diet should contain something from all the food groups such as fruits, vegetables, grains, dairy products, fish, meat, carbohydrates and fats.

Expected mother's diet should include approximately:

- **20%** of fruits and vegetables
- **50%** of cereals, whole grain breads, pasta or rice
- **15%** of dairy products such as milk, cheese and yogurt
- **15%** of poultry, fish, meat, nuts, peas, and beans

It is very important for expected mother to drink plenty of water, juices and milk. Read over the chapter "Water" in this book for all explanations and suggestions.

There are some _vitamins and minerals that are absolutely essential during pregnancy:_ **iron**, **folic acid**, **protein**, **zinc** and **calcium**.

Dietary iron

Dietary iron is a crucial part of red blood cells, which transport oxygen throughout the body and supply nutrients to the placenta.

Good sources of iron:

Red meat – especially liver; **poultry** – especially dark meat; **fish** – tuna, salmon, sardines and any type of shellfish; **eggs**; **leafy green vegetables** – spinach, kale, collards and broccoli; **legumes** – beans and peas; **grains** – wheat and oats, whole wheat bread; **soy products** – tofu and soymilk.

Iron is more easily absorbed if it is taken with vitamin C – either as a supplement or in citrus fruit or juice. Iron is also absorbed better when animal sources of iron are eaten with green leafy vegetables. On the contrary, tea and coffee can interfere with the body's absorption of iron. In addition, consumption of dietary iron should be spread throughout the day, ideally in three or more doses, because the human body is not capable of absorbing large amounts of iron in a short time.

Folic acid

Folic acid plays a large role in cell growth and development, as well as tissue formation. It is used by the body to make new cells, and it is used to make the extra blood the body needs during pregnancy. It is also crucial in the development of DNA. It is especially important to have enough of folic acid in the body one month before conception and during early pregnancy. The absence of folic acid increases the possibility of various birth defects, including neural tube defects; so expected mothers should pay attention.

Good sources of folic acid:

Dark green leafy vegetables – lettuce, spinach, kale, mustard greens, collard, and turnip greens; *fruits high in folic acid* – strawberries, grapefruit, mandarin and other oranges, orange juice, kiwi, honeydew, cantaloupe, mango, papaya, and tangerine. Folic acid can also be found in broccoli, green peas, asparagus, pastas, rice, wheat germ, dried beans, and fortified grains.

Protein

Protein is the basis of all new tissues created during pregnancy. The amino acids, which make up protein, also form building blocks of mother's body's cells, which in turn also form building blocks of baby's body too. Protein is also required for the placenta, amniotic tissues, and maternal tissues. In addition, a woman's blood volume doubles during pregnancy, and protein is needed to produce new blood cells. Protein is also utilized to produce breast milk and nourish the growing baby. **Pregnant women need about 60 – 70 grams of protein each day**, which is about 20% more than a norm prior to the pregnancy. *For suggested sources of protein, read the chapter "Proteins" above.*

Zinc

Zinc is a critical nutrient to have during pregnancy, as it *plays an important role in all phases of growth* of the fetus. It stabilizes the genetic code in each cell so that growth goes as planned. It is also a component of insulin, which helps to regulate the glucose needed by baby, and much more. Zinc is also necessary for the formation of sperm, ovum, ovulation and fertilization. Zinc deficiency can result in pregnancy-related toxemia, spontaneous abortion, premature or extended delivery and prolonged labor, and even some birth defects. *We discussed zinc in great detail in chapter "Zinc", where sources of zinc are described*, so my advice is to read it over. **The daily requirement for zinc during pregnancy is 13-15 milligrams**, but a higher dose may be needed. Women should consult their physician before taking zinc or any other supplement during pregnancy.

Calcium

Calcium is important during pregnancy because your developing baby needs it to grow strong bones and teeth, nerves, a healthy heart, muscles, also to develop normal heart rhythm and blood clotting abilities. Calcium can also keep the blood pressure normal, and may reduce the risk of pre-term delivery. *If you don't get enough calcium during pregnancy, your bones will become a source of calcium for your baby, which may weaken your bones in the future.* Before, during, and after pregnancy expected mother needs up to 1,000 mg of calcium a day or 1300 mg for women under age 19. *For suggested sources of calcium, please read the chapter "Calcium" above in the book.*

To be avoided during pregnancy:

◆ *Raw meat* such as uncooked or undercooked beef, eggs, poultry or seafood (especially raw shellfish) because it may contain harmful bacteria and bacterial toxins

◆ *Fish with high levels of mercury* such as tuna, shark, swordfish, king mackerel, and tilefish, may result in developmental delays and even brain damage

◆ *Fish exposed to industrial and other pollutants* from contaminated lakes and rivers

◆ *Un-pasteurized milk* and any *un-pasteurized cheeses* because they may contain bacteria that can infect the baby and the mother

◆ *Foods with large amounts of vitamin A,* such as liver and cod liver oil, should be avoided during pregnancy because it may cause damage to the embryo and should be eaten on an occasional basis only

◆ *Alcohol* may very negatively affect the baby's development in many ways, therefore should be completely avoided

◆ *Caffeine drinks* should be significantly reduced or better-off completely avoided, especially in the first three months of pregnancy. As I described it in the chapter "Water", caffeine reduces the amount of water in the body, which is absolutely crucial for the baby's development. Caffeine also flashes-out necessary calcium

◆ *Smoking* is one of most damaging things expected mother can do. *Most children whose mother has been smoking during pregnancy gain less in height than their piers*

When child is born

First several years of life are crucial to a child's future final height.
To put it simply, a child that gets all needed vitamins and minerals
and does not get any major diseases during infancy will grow taller
than a child who does not have all that, sometimes much taller.

My main suggestion to parents of newborn: *please try your best
to breastfeed your child for at least 5 – 6 months.* You will give the
most important basis for good health for the rest of your child's life.
Nothing can replace breast milk. It is the optimal source of nutrition
during infancy, including the best possible source of zinc, which is
also absorbed much better than from any other sources.

> Just for your information, breastfeeding lowers the risk of
> infections and allergies, even into adulthood, and may boost
> brain development early in life. Also, breastfed infants may be less
> likely to grow into overweight children than formula-fed babies.

Even best prepared baby formula does not provide most of the disease-
protective factors that are present in breast milk. Statistically, formula-
fed infants are generally sicker and get sick more often. They are *three
to four times* more likely to have diarrhea or an ear infection, and *ten
times* more likely to get complications from bacterial infections.

Breastfeeding is also great for mother's health, and one of the main
benefits of it is significantly decreased risk of breast cancer and ovarian
cancer in the future.

Another interesting fact: a new study examined siblings who were
breastfed and bottle-fed, and found that for each additional month
a baby is breastfed, their high school GPA increases. Therefore, if
you breastfeed your baby for even just three months, his or her
future GPA is likely to go up and the probability of attending college
increases too.

There are many other benefits to breastfeeding that are just beyond the scope of this book. But in regards to the body growth, **breastfeeding during infancy does increase the future final height of a person**. No studied have found so far that breastfeeding directly affects body growth, in many cases formula-fed babies tend to grow taller in first years of life, even in their teens. However, statistics show that those who were breastfed, eventually overgrow their peers, especially during last years of their body's growth. The explanation to this phenomenon is simple: *breastfed children grow healthier and don't get sick as often and as serious as artificially-fed children*. As we already know – healthier children's final height is almost always greater; therefore breastfed children have greater chance to be taller.

As for other recommendations for parents of a small child, it is very important for a child to be checked with a pediatrician on a constant basis, and follow all doctor's recommendations, including a child's diet. Let me stress-out one more time that **wide variety of vitamins and minerals is especially essential for our youngest loved ones**.

If you want your young child to grow at full potential, it is also extremely important to make sure a child is **physically active every day**. Exercises should be performed from child's first day of life. Ask a doctor how to do it, and never forget doing it.

Children massages are very important as well, especially for infants, to ensure their complete development and to stimulate their growth. Massage points to stimulate the release of growth hormone are recommended in the "Stimulating reflex zones" section of a chapter "Growth Hormone", can also apply for infants. Also, you will find some suggestions for baby massage the chapter "Massage" of this book. You should understand that *massage of infants has to be done with extreme care and knowledge*, and should be carried by a professional. Parents can also perform some basics, but must learn first from a doctor or a professional children masseuse.

The rule about water/salt balance we have learned in chapters "Water" and "Salt" applies to small children as well. I strongly suggest reading those chapters again and follow all recommendations there. *Water is absolutely essential for everybody, especially for younger children. It plays very important role in child's development and growth.*

Just as older children and adults, younger children must get some direct Sun exposure, preferably every day. As we discussed it thoroughly in the chapter "Affects of Sunlight", exposure to the Sun is necessary for the health of every living cell in our body, for healthy bones, and for the energy we need to function fully. You should definitely be extra careful to overexpose your child to the ultraviolet light of the Sun, and the best way to do that is getting the child out into the sun only couple hours after sunrise and before sunset.

If you are an adult and still want to be taller

If you are an adult and did not bother to read this entire book, let me point out that even though this book is written for our younger generation, **practically everything in here will apply for an adult as well**. If you would like to be healthier, I strongly recommend reading the entire book because *all of the information you will find in the book is important to know at any age*. I'm positive you will find a lot of important details you never knew. Moreover, **a lot of information in in this book you will not find anywhere else**.

Well, there is *bad news* and there is *good news*. The bad news is that if your growth plates had been completely fused, your bones cannot grow. The good news is that you can still increase your height by 1% – 3% of your total body length. How is it possible? By *improving your posture and improving the health of your spinal discs*.

Yes, your height will increase simply by improving your posture. I don't need to explain why as it is simple logic. To accomplish that read my recommendation from the chapter "Your Posture", also you will get much better posture if you will follow the entire exercise program in this book (*of course, you will gain much more benefits from this exercise program than just improved posture and height*).

Regarding the improving the health of your spinal discs, let's get into more details about this, as it is very important to understand.

Let me start with an interesting fact: astronauts temporarily become on average two inches (5 cm) taller when they are in space for over

12 weeks. That is why space suits are made two inches taller than the astronaut's normal height. How does it happen?

> *All of us on Earth are under constant pressure from gravity, which presses us hard to the ground compressing our entire body when we are in vertical position. Under this constant pressure our skeleton's weakest parts, cartilages between joints, are squeezed and shrink. Most cartilages affected by gravitation are in the spine. These cartilage pads, called intervertebral discs or spinal discs, separate bones of the spine forming cushions that keep those bones from grinding against each other and making the spine flexible, also acting as shock absorbers. There are 23 of them; each is about a quarter to three quarters of an inch thick, and all of them make up about one-third of the length of the spine. They compress when weight is put on them and spring back when the weight is removed.*

Therefore the astronaut's height gain in space is a natural reaction to the loss of gravity's pull on the spine, which allows the spine to lengthen.

As we discussed earlier in the book, the same happens to us at night when gravity does not prevent the spine from lengthening when we lay down. As you understand this, you should also understand that *if all those intervertebral discs would become permanently thicker, your spine would permanently lengthen, and your height would increase.* How do we permanently increase thickness of intervertebral discs naturally? To answer that we should understand what these discs are made of and how they can expand or shrink.

Spinal discs are composed of a tough outer wall and a softer, pliable inner core. Imagine it as a car tire with gel inside instead of air, where the tire rubber is the outer wall of a disc that is thick and multilayered to resist wear and tear, and the gel inside of the tire is the inner core of a disc which is moist, much more flexible and full of necessary nutrients. Just like with a tire, spinal disc is larger when inflated and smaller when deflated. *For a spinal disc to be inflated, its inner core should soak up nutrient rich fluid*. This is where it gets interesting and very important to understand.

Before we go on, let me point out that height increase as a result of inflated spinal discs is relatively small and unimportant benefit in comparison to true importance of healthy spinal discs. *Healthy discs should be thick (inflated) and flexible to make them easily bend, twist and be good shock absorbers. Unhealthy discs* are thin (deflated), stiff, hard, and have more chance to be injured. Usually young and growing person rarely have such a problem, which is why we did not thoroughly discuss this previously in the book. As we age however, the discs naturally tend to dehydrate and shrink. Over time gravity constantly compresses and flattens them, which prevents much-needed oxygen and nutrients from entering, making outer layers of the disc to soften. This allows the disc to become injured or diseased, often leading to degenerative disc disease. Such condition can squeeze nerves that are running through the spine, disconnecting signals between the brain and many organs in the body leading to numerous problems outside of the spine.

The constant internal disc pressure consistently pushes the fluid out of the disc, making it difficult to suck-in new fluid with its much-needed oxygen and nutrients. So, how does nutrient rich fluid gets inside of the disc inner core to keep it healthy, in other words – how do spine discs get inflated?

Discs have no blood supply; therefore, unlike the rest of the body, they cannot receive nutrients delivered by blood. The discs soak up their nutrient rich fluid **only** *through spinal joint movements and while at rest*. This brings us to the main conclusion: **if you rarely exercise or stretch your spine and don't give it enough rest, spine discs will eventually degenerate and shrink, making you shorter and venerable to many diseases**. Also, *if your body does not get enough water and necessary nutrients, it significantly adds to the problem*.

To keep your spine healthy and to maximize your height for the rest of your life, you always need to supply your body with *right nutrients, enough water,* and ensure that your spine gets *proper physical workout,* as well as *enough rest* every single day.

Most of the **nutrients** for the healthy spine discs and for all other connective tissue in our skeleton have already discussed earlier in the book in full detail, and I suggest going over with all of them. Most important for the health of bone and connective tissue are these nutrients: vitamin – C, D, E, K, all of the B vitamins, especially B6, and the minerals – calcium, magnesium, zinc, copper, and manganese.

We have discussed the importance of **water** very throughway in this book (see Chapter "Water"); therefore you should already know that drinking enough water is also essential for healthy spinal discs because the water is the discs' main substance, especially in the inner core. Please read chapter "Water" to remind yourself what water to drink, how to drink it correctly, how much, and when, as it is one of the most important pieces of information in this book.

Let's discuss **proper physical workout** for the healthy spine. As we've just learned, without it your spinal discs will slowly but surely shrink or deflate. Even when your body has all necessary nutrients and enough water, *without proper movements and stretches, those nutrients and water will not be able to get into spinal discs, leaving them deflated and unhealthy.* So, what physical workout is proper for the spine? Interestingly enough, such exercise routine is fully described above in this book in "Spinal column workout" section of the chapter "Physical Exercise", and designed to get every disc of the spine involved, from top to the bottom. Those exercises are exactly what I recommend you to do. Of course, first consult your doctor, especially when you had any injuries or problems with the spine, because certain exercises will be very good for some spine conditions, and possibly harmful for others.

Go over the exercise routine described in the chapter "Physical Exercise", but let me point out *most important points for an adult to keep in mind*.

♦ First of all, everything that you do physically has to be gradual. Never start or end any exercise with sudden spike in activity or sudden stop, just take your time and take it easy because you will make more harm to your body otherwise.

♦ Allow physical stress only once or twice a day, and only for several seconds, sometimes up to 30 – 60 seconds, depending on your physical health. It is a good way to boost the growth hormone release, which is needed at any age. The rest of the exercise routine should be performed in relaxed state.

♦ Do not make any fast or sudden moves, especially when you get your spine involved. If you do, prepare yourself by worming-up first.

♦ Follow entire routine, including every part of the spinal column – neck, upper, lower, and lumbar spinal cords. Do not leave anything out because every part of our spine is very important.

♦ A very important part of your exercise routine should be stretching, and a chin-up bar should be your best friend for that. Simple hanging from the bar while being relaxed will do it, but if you will follow other suggestions from the section "Chin-up Bar Workout" in the chapter "Physical Exercise" – even better. When we hang, the spine gently extends, creating a vacuum inside of spinal discs, allowing discs to absorb the needed moisture with nutrients and oxygen from surrounding blood vessels.

♦ Another good equipment to have is inversion table, which hangs you upside down. Its benefit compared to hanging from the bar is that the neck spinal cord is also being decompressed. There are other benefits to hanging upside down, but you should know that it could also result in some unpleasant side effects including headaches or bleeding into your eyes. And, it could even worsen your back problem if you have such. Therefore, definitely ask your doctor before using such equipment.

The last factor affecting your spine, **enough rest**, is not the least important. I'm sure you will like the suggestion to give your spine more rest. Who wouldn't? Yes, try to lay down for at least a few minutes during the day, and have enough sleep at night, at least 8 hours, on a firm orthopedic mattress, with a small pillow or no pillow. For more suggestions about proper sleep, read the chapter "Sleep" above.

You should also understand that lying down is not the only option to give your spine more rest. Releasing stress from your back will also give your spine more rest. Using correct posture and keeping your spine in alignment are the most important things you can do for your back. The way you stand or sit, the way you bend or lift, make a big difference. Read about how to keep the correct posture in the chapter "Your Posture". When you bend or pick up something heavy, always bend both of your legs, do not bend your spine.

When holding something, always hold it as close as possible to your body, trying to keep your spine up straight. Often switch your hands or shoulders when holding something heavy. Always use lumbar support when sitting, especially at work or in the car.

Another important way to give your spine more rest is by trying to keep your muscles relaxed at all times. When your muscles are stiff, your spine will be under additional pressure, even when you are lying down. Great ways to relax your muscles are good massage (of course), relaxation exercises and deep breathing exercises (see chapter "Breathing").

Keep in mind that too much rest for the spine is also not good. On top of exercises that I recommend, try to keep your spine and neck flexing and bending all the time, even slightly. Don't let you spine to be still for long, keep it moving. Even though we are discussing spine only in this chapter, don't forget to keep you entire body moving, and *the entire exercise program in this book is actually great for any age, not only for young people*.

Another big factor affecting the compression and health of the spine is overweight, especially with abdominal fat. Not surprisingly, if you've read this book entirely, you already know many factors that can affect a person's weight safely and naturally.

How To Succeed

Now, my dear friend, you know almost everything about human growth and how to increase it (except last little secret later in this chapter). Even though this book is relatively small because I tried to keep it as short and as easy for you to understand as possible, it does cover a lot of information and a lot of secrets you won't find anywhere else today. I'm sure some of this information was overwhelming for you, which is understandable. If you did not understand something, read it again and again until you do, because all of the information I included in this book is important if you are serious about increasing your height.

I wrote this book for you, my young feller, as well as for my own beautiful children (I hope they will follow my advices as well). Everything I gave you in this book came not only from many years of experience and serious research, but also from my heart. I truly want you to succeed in your desire to accomplish your great goal, and I know – you can do it.

As I mentioned number of times throughout the book, what you have learned here not only will help you in your quest to grow taller, but will also give you basics for your health, strength, and all your other future accomplishments for the rest of your life. Don't just keep it as the knowledge, use it and you will not regret it, I promise.

Don't wait for tomorrow to start following suggestions in this book, start today and keep it going one day at a time. All the suggestions I gave in the book are easy to follow; even food intake suggestions that seemed overwhelming at first site have a lot of options and flexibility, and comes down basically to eating wide variety of healthy food in suggested proportions. If you don't see expected results soon enough, don't be discouraged, and also understand that *if you follow this program, you are doing much more for yourself then just trying to increase your height,* so don't think that you have wasted anything, you only gained. Just be patient, and you will succeed. Keep in mind that *it takes time for your body to react to the changes in your activities.*

Are you ready to start? If so, the first thing you can do is to measure your height on the wall, doorframe, or any other vertical object that you are not planning to remove or paint for the next few years. You can ask your parents or your friends to hold any object that has a 90-degree angle (it can be a book) on top of your head, while you are standing straight against this vertical object. Mark your height in pen with a small line and write the date of measurement under this line. This should be the only measurement that you will take during the first year. Don't check your results during this year, just do everything you need to do, and you already know it all after reading this book. *Check your height in a year from now,* and you will likely to find yourself pleasantly surprised.

There are many important secrets revealed in this book, but one that I reserved for the last may be more important than all of the above combined. It is the formula to accomplish anything you may desire, including increasing height. We went trough basics of this secret throughout this book, so I hope you will understand and appreciate the power of its simple formula. Here it is: **smile + straight posture = good mood = any goals accomplished**

Yes, simply smiling and keeping a good posture will improve your mood which will truly do wonders. When you are constantly and passionately trying to look as a happy person, you will become a happy person! Do you think I'm exaggerating the power of a "happy person" feeling? This feeling alone can cure practically any disease and lay the road to your success in anything that you do. True happiness comes when you create it in your mind first, not when events around you will make you happy. Smile my friend with confidence, don't be afraid to be different if no one else smiles around you, widen your shoulders, keep your spine and head straight and hold it that way for as long as you can. As you do that, *make a firm command in your mind to what you want to accomplish. If you are persistent enough, passionate about your goal, and patient enough, this command will materialize.* That is the law on which human civilization is built. With this law there are no limits on what you can accomplish.

If you don't keep your posture straight, if your face is usually grim, don't even dream to have any significant results from this book. *Don't wait for something good to make a smile, make a smile to create something good.*

Smile and you will stand tall regardless of your height!

When you say: "I hope I will ..." – you become a beggar;

When you say: "I definitely will ..." – you become a winner!

All winners won believing in their victory.

Their thoughts of victory materialized, so will yours.

Please visit the discussion forum at
www.grow-taller.com/forum *where many follow-ers of this program are sharing their experiences and results with each other*

If you have any questions or comments on this book, please email at: **info@grow-taller.com**

If you like this book and think that your friend will benefit from it too, please let your friend know

If you would like to earn money by selling this book, please go to **www.grow-taller.com/affiliates** *for instructions*